"Saki Santorelli's words have the gentle strength of a bird's wings, beating softly as they gradually bear us aloft. Brave, beautiful, and disturbing, his book reminds us of the healing that conventional Western medicine has all but forgotten. I wish it had been available when I was in medical school."

MARK EPSTEIN, M.D., author of
Going to Pieces Without Falling Apart

"In prose, poetry, and poignant case examples, Saki evokes for us the mutuality of the healing relationship and reclaims for medicine and all who work within it the wisdom and power of its lineage. *Heal Thy Self* is a clear mirror in which we can find that freedom which is at the heart of all authentic healing and through it reconsecrate ourselves to our work and to our lives."

RACHEL NAOMI REMEN, M.D.,
author of *Kitchen Table Wisdom*

"A simply beautiful book. A full body/mind/heart contact between that which is healing within and that, a bit further in, which promotes that healing. A most necessary book for any medical student or healing library."

STEPHEN LEVINE, author of *A Year to Live*

"This is a remarkable, helpful book. Its genuine and warmhearted teaching gives us a real glimpse of the path of healing. Recommended to everyone, new or old, on the path of life."

CHARLOTTE JOKO BECK, author of *Everyday Zen*

"Saki Santorelli shows the fruit of his dedicated effort in presenting mindfulness as not just the stuff of meditation retreats and stress reduction seminars. His accounts of everything from counseling a depressed woman to _____ _____ _____ year-old daughter encounter a homeless perso_____ _____ _____ sic truths of our lives. It is hon_____

SHARON SALZBERG, a_____ _____ _____ rld

Heal Thy Self

Lessons on
Mindfulness in Medicine

Dear Christina,

I was touched deeply by your being touched so powerfully in regards to your sense of calling. I wish you well in your journey.

Saki Santorelli

Warmly

THREE RIVERS PRESS · NEW YORK

Saki Santorelli 2/28/2010

Grateful acknowledgment is made to the following for permission to reprint previously published material: "The Devil's Sooty Brother" from *The Complete Fairy Tales of the Brothers Grimm* by Jack Zipes, translation copyright © 1987 by Jack Zipes, used by permission of Bantam Books, a division of Bantam Doubleday Dell Publishing Group. Poem #33 from *The Kabir Book: Versions by Robert Bly,* copyright © 1971, 1977 by Robert Bly, reprinted by permission of Beacon Press, Boston. Excerpt from *Times Alone: Fourteen Poems from Antonio Machado,* translated by Robert Bly, copyright © 1983 by Robert Bly, used by permission of the author. #76 and #78 from *Tao Te Ching by Lao Tzu, A New English Version,* with foreword and notes by Stephen Mitchell, translation copyright © 1988 by Stephen Mitchell, reprinted by permission of HarperCollins Publishers, Inc. "In Blackwater Woods" from *American Primitive* by Mary Oliver, copyright © 1983 by Mary Oliver (first appeared in *Yankee* magazine), used by permission of Little, Brown and Company. Excerpt from "The Journey" from *Dream Work* by Mary Oliver, copyright © 1986 by Mary Oliver, used by permission of the author and Grove/Atlantic, Inc. "The Summer Day" from *House of Light* by Mary Oliver, copyright © 1990 by Mary Oliver, reprinted by permission of Beacon Press, Boston. Excerpt of Rumi's "Childhood Friends" from *Delicious Laughter,* translated by Coleman Barks, copyright © 1990, and Rumi's "The Guest-House" and "The Pick-Axe" from *Say I Am You,* translated by John Moyne and Coleman Barks, copyright © 1994 by Coleman Barks, both reprinted by permission of Maypop Books, Athens, Georgia. Rumi's "Two Kinds of Intelligence" from *This Longing,* quatrain #158 and an excerpt of "Unmarked Boxes" from *Open Secret,* both translated by Coleman Barks and John Moyne and used by permission of Threshold Books, 139 Main Street, Brattleboro, VT 05301. Poem by Izumi Shikibu from *The Ink Dark Moon: Love Poems by Ono no Komachi and Izumi Shikibu* by Jane Hirshfield with Mariko Aratani, copyright © 1986, 1987, 1988, 1989, 1990 by Jane Hirshfield, reprinted by permission of Vintage Books, a division of Random House, Inc.

Foreword copyright © 1999 by Jon Kabat-Zinn, Ph.D.
Text copyright © 1999 by Saki Santorelli

Published in the United States by Three Rivers Press, an imprint of the Crown Publishing Group, a division of Random House, Inc., New York. Originally published in hardcover in the United States by Bell Tower, an imprint of the Crown Publishing Group, a division of Random House, Inc., New York, in 1999. First paperback edition published in 2000.

www.crownpublishing.com

Three Rivers Press and the Tugboat design are registered trademarks of Random House, Inc.

Printed in the United States of America
Design by LYNNE AMFT

Library of Congress Cataloging-in-Publication Data
Santorelli, Saki.
Heal thy self : lessons on mindfulness in medicine / Saki
Santorelli.— 1st ed.
Includes bibliographical references.
1. Stress management.   2. Healing.   3. Meditation.   4. Attention.   5. Medical personnel and
patient.   I. Title.
RA785.S28   1999
155.9'042—dc21   98-34968
CIP

ISBN 0-609-80504-5

10 9

For Rachmana, Chalice, and Felice—
may we continue to unfold in the presence of one another.
For my parents, Rose and Fred—
thank you for enormous love freely given.

Out beyond ideas of wrongdoing and rightdoing,
there is a field. I'll meet you there.

When the soul lies down in that grass,
the world is too full to talk about.
Ideas, language, even the phrase each other
doesn't make any sense.

RUMI
Quatrain #158 from *Open Secret*

Contents

Acknowledgments

RECOGNITION OF THE interdependent nature of our existence is easily overlooked in the press of everyday life. In my attempts to honor the actuality of this interconnectedness, writing these acknowledgments has been instructional, a powerful reminder to me of the scores of people who have contributed directly and indirectly to this book. I wish to bow to the force of their presence in my life.

I thank Jon Kabat-Zinn, Ph.D., the founder of the Stress Reduction Clinic and the executive director of the Center for Mindfulness in Medicine, Health Care, and Society at the University of Massachusetts Medical School. Since 1981, he has been my boss, mentor, colleague, teaching partner, and most fundamentally a friend and fellow companion on the inner journey from which this book has arisen. Trained in both the basic and contemplative sciences, his commitment to the joining of "inner and outer," "spirit and matter," "form and formlessness," has had a profound effect in my life and in the worlds of medicine and health care. For his vision, wisdom, wit, and friendship, I am forever grateful.

I wish to thank Judith K. Ockene, Ph.D., director of the division of Preventive and Behavioral Medicine in the Department of Medicine at the University of Massachusetts Medical School, for her encouragement and open-mindedness. I have learned much from her during the last fifteen years and she has given me ample room to grow into what is mine to do.

I thank the 1,400 physicians in central Massachusetts and the surrounding New England region who have referred their patients to the Stress Reduction Clinic and the far smaller cadre of these physicians with whom I work more closely at UMass Memorial Health Care. In particular, I wish to express my gratitude to John

Moynahan, M.D.; John Zawacki, M.D.; Sarah Stone, M.D.; David Clive, M.D.; Ira Ockene, M.D.; David Giansiracusa, M.D.; David Hatem, M.D.; Ed Landeau, M.D.; Andy Cohen, M.D.; Ilia Shlimak, M.D.; Bill Damon, M.D.; Lynn Manfred, M.D.; and Mai-Lan Rogoff, M.D. Their dedication to educating the next generation of physicians, to engaging in patient-centered care, and going the extra mile in the service of those whom they serve remains for me a wellspring of inspiration and a quiet source of pride. In addition, I wish to express my gratitude to Marty Young, Ph.D.; Majorie Clay, Ph.D.; Michael Wertheimer, M.D.; and H. Brownell Wheeler, M.D., for their presence and support.

My teaching colleagues in the Stress Reduction Clinic have been unflagging sources of inspiration and encouragement. I cannot imagine a finer group of people to work with. I wish to thank Ferris Urbanowski, M.A., for her unbounded radiance and her enthusiasm and willingness to read and reread drafts of the manuscript—and, most of all, for her unwavering attention to and insights about the relational aspects of mindfulness and the healing encounter. I thank Elana Rosenbaum, L.I.C.S.W., for her huge heart, undying courage, and capacity to stand inside the truth of her own experience; Pamela Erdmann, M.Ed., for her honesty, integrity, and dedication to teaching mindfulness in the Massachusetts prison system; Florence Meyer, M.A., M.S., for her listening, her embodiment of spaciousness and safety so beautifully evidenced in the classroom, and for her detailed feedback about an early draft of the manuscript; Melissa Blacker for the depth of her Zen practice and its sensitive, playful expression in her work; Fernando de Torrijos for his compassionate heart, gentlemanly manner, and breadth of knowledge about the contemplative traditions, and more so, for he and Melissa's shared commitment to bringing the heart of mindfulness practice to low-income, medically underserved, inner-city residents in Worcester, Massachusetts.

My deep appreciation goes to Larry Horwitz, M.B.A., for his dharmically oriented organizational acumen and for our evolving friendship; to Anne Skillings, M.S., for her quick mind, long-standing attention to our research, and capacity to skillfully play a hundred roles; to Leigh Emery, R.N., M.S., for her administrative vision and the richness of her poetry; and to Michael Bratt, Ph.D., for his enthusiasm for mindfulness practice, his dedication to the clinic's research endeavors, and his capacity to bring together a research team. I give thanks to Carol Lewis, Sylvia Ciarlo, Roberta Lewis, Leslie Lynch, Norma Rosiello, and, most recently, Jean Baril and Carmen Torres for taking responsibility for the day-to-day operation of the clinic while actively participating in shaping the unfolding vision of the Center for Mindfulness in Medicine, Health Care, and Society.

This book would not have been possible without the ten thousand patients who have participated in the Stress Reduction Clinic since 1979 and who decided to roll up their sleeves and take up the practice of mindfulness as a way of learning to work with stress, pain, and illness. Their presence in my life has been nothing short of transformative. I pray that I have done them justice in attempting to capture the actuality of their lives and their efforts.

I am indebted to my wife, Rachmana, and my two daughters, Chalice and Felice. While I was writing this book, they generously offered me the gifts of time and space as well as keen eyes and an uncanny capacity for directness and clarity. Their support and love are a blessing to me. I thank my parents, Rose and Fred Santorelli, for all that they have given to me over the years and my sister, Rosanne, for her ongoing efforts to meet the world through her heart. On the other side of the family, my in-laws, Doug and Pearl Robinson, have taught me much. Pearl's persistent intention to steer her own life course has helped me to better understand some of my patients' strong desires to do the same; and Doug's quick smile, quiet knowing, and innate sense of telling the right story at just the right time are qualities to which I aspire.

I thank Stephan Rechtschaffen, M.D., for his friendship and for offering me a clinical position in the nascent field of mind-body medicine back in 1980. Many thanks to Monica Faulkner for her early encouragement and steadfast support. I am grateful for the friendship of David Weinberg, a fine mindfulness-based stress reduction teacher living in Berkeley, California, and his wife, Karen Elliot, who provided me a warm and caring shelter during a particularly difficult period of my life while I was writing this book. Many thanks to Bob Stahl, Ph.D., Patrick Thornton, Ph.D., and Amy Saltzman, M.D., for helping to anchor, with maturity and mastery, the unfolding of a mindfulness-based stress reduction teachers network in the San Francisco Bay Area. My gratitude to Elizabeth Lesser for the sweetness of our friendship and our teaching forays into "quiet mind/open heart."

I wish to thank the thousands of health professionals who have participated in our Professional Education and Development Programs at the clinic or who have attended our residential retreat/training programs in different parts of the country. The presence, energy, and courage you directed toward looking into and speaking openly about your own woundedness, about your original calling to be of service in medicine and health care, and your longing for more authentic, less time-bound relationships with your patients have become an enfolded part of my own life. The traces of your presence run like a river through this book.

In a similar vein, I offer thanks to the first- and second-year medical students with whom I have worked closely during the last twelve years. Your vigilant attention to what first called you to medicine and the anxiety, pain, and indignation you've expressed when facing the possibility of having that calling diminished in the rush of medical education is a mark of your dignity. I am heartened that you honor your calling in such a manner; your dedication is a consistent reminder to me of my own vocation.

With deep respect and appreciation I wish to acknowledge the work of the mythologist Karl Kerényi, who has reinvested contemporary medicine with the archetypal truth of the Greek myth of Chiron—the wounded healer. Likewise, I thank the Jungian psychiatrist Adolph Guggenbühl-Craig for his deep insights into the healing relationship when framed within the polarities of the *wounded healer* and the *healthy patient* existing within each of us. Together, their seminal insights substantiated in the day-to-day world of clinical care, when joined with mindfulness practice, are some of the seeds from which this book has blossomed.

I thank professors Gerald Weinstein, Jack Wideman, Patricia Griffith, and Alfred Alschuler for being ahead of their time while I was a graduate student in the School of Education at the University of Massachusetts in Amherst. My appreciation goes out to the poet Robert Bly, from whom I first heard a few lines of the Brothers Grimm story "The Devil's Sooty Brother."

I offer gratitude to Swami Satchidananda and profound thanks to the Sufi teachers Hazrat Inayat Khan, Vilayat Inayat Kahn, and Taj Glantz, as well as to mindfulness meditation teachers Larry Rosenberg, Corrado Pensa, Sharon Salzberg, Christina Feldman, Kamala Masters, Vimalo Kulbarz, and Thich Nhat Hanh. What I have learned from each of them is at the core of this book.

My editor, Toinette Lippe, has been nothing less than extraordinary. She understood this book from the beginning. Both challenging and supportive, her editorial skills coupled with her own grounding in meditative practice brought a discerning crispness and a spacious acceptance to the process that enabled us to work well together. I am happy to have been led to her and to the Random House/Bell Tower family. Special thanks to Mary Schuck, the artist who designed the cover; to Lynne Amft, who designed the interior; to Andrea Peabbles, the production editor who guided the book to completion; and to John Sharp, the production manager who oversaw manufacturing.

Foreword

ON THE EVE OF THE TWENTIETH anniversary of the Stress Reduction Clinic, I am moved by a profound sense of gratitude and pleasure to see this book by my longtime colleague, heart friend, and dharma brother Saki Santorelli emerge in the world, giving as it does a new, radiant, and powerful voice to the work that transpires in the clinic and to the deeper underlying principles and practices that inform and sustain it. I am speaking of the work of mindfulness in all its exquisite simplicity, its vast complexity, and its infinite ramifications of texture, tone, and potential. As you will see within these pages, mindfulness is both an inner and an outer engagement, one that is critical, I believe, to the maintaining and the furthering of what is best in us as individuals and as a society.

We have probably all had the experience of not being seen or heard by a doctor when we presented a problem or concern; of coming away feeling disregarded, unmet, and therefore unfulfilled in the encounter, regardless of the doctor's degree of technical proficiency. At the turn of both century and millennium, medicine is coming to learn that this is no longer acceptable as a norm, and doctors are seeing more and more how a lack of full presence on their part can have deleterious consequences not only for their patients but for their own ultimate well-being as well. And when we ourselves become patients, we are now as a rule far less passive, far more informed, and far more desirous of partnership in the healing process than in past decades. Medical schools have understood this message, and doctors are currently being trained in how to be with patients, in how to listen, in how not to hide emotionally, in how to help mobilize the inner resources of their patients for learning, growing, and healing. While much progress has been made, there is still a long way to go in the rehumanizing of medicine. My hope is that this book will contribute in a major way to the furthering and deepening of this process, and will become standard reading for all medical students and health professionals in training. Saki is intimately engaged in this education through his work with medical students, beautifully captured here, and of course, in his work with the people who are referred by their medical doctors to the clinic, where they get the opportunity to participate in their own health care and healing in extraordinary and unimagined ways.

The stories in this book, taken together, have the deepest of implications for the larger world of medicine and health care and the mutual relationship between caregivers and patients and its potential to further bidirectional learning, growing, healing, and transformation in us all. The stories beg to be pondered with great care and attentiveness. That should be no problem, because Saki's mind and voice within these pages are nothing less than electrifying, at times bordering on Old Testament prophet, at times much more embodying the respectful sensitivity of the lover or the pain and embarrassment of being trapped by one's own inevitable limitations and fears and impulses to hide. I have personally experienced the emotional impact of this book firsthand as a reader and I have also witnessed the effect of Saki's writing on hundreds of health professionals when he has read from his book during workshops we conduct together—at least a quarter of the audience is soon sobbing, the others sitting in stunned silence, rocked by its emotional power and its implications.

Saki speaks with a unique voice in this book. The closest I can come to describing it is to say that, even though it is prose, in its cadence, its images, and its spiritual and emotional impact, it echoes the writing of Rumi, the thirteenth-century Sufi poet and sage from whom Saki draws so freely in weaving the formative themes of this book. And yet in content and appeal, it is totally contemporary. It speaks in straightforward and commonsensical ways to what is deepest and best and most hidden in all of us by virtue of our humanness, to that which most wants to emerge into the light of day in spite of our fears and our tendency to live in our heads more than in the fullness of our entire being: mind *and* body, head *and* heart, body *and* soul; to that which we sometimes can only hear or see if we learn to dwell in silence and in stillness from time to time, inside and underneath the incessant activity of the mind and the body.

Heal Thy Self is a book of interwoven themes that form one seamless whole out of which emerges a clear and compelling tableau of human dignity, human suffering, human uplift, and what might be possible when the whole is held in awareness and we learn to stand within the actuality of what is. It is about meditation when life is breathed into it, and about life when meditation is breathed into it. It is about the healing relationship between people brought together for that purpose, and it is about the possibilities of a healing relationship within oneself and in one's family, at any age, facing any condition or situation. It weaves with honesty and without inflation or romanticism the experience of our patients going through the eight-week-long stress reduction clinic program with Saki's own experience as teacher, guide, meditator, health professional, and family member. It brings out with utter authenticity and accuracy the heart of what transpires in our patients and in ourselves as instructors as we walk this path together. This is in itself a huge accomplishment and a major contribution to the expanding understanding of what is truly meant and promised by an integrative medicine, by mind/body medicine, by a participatory medicine, and ultimately simply by *good* medicine.

In an earlier incarnation, this book was to be called *Shattered But Still Whole,* and those words convey one extremely moving thread that holds this tapestry together and makes it so compelling. Saki asks over and over again, in many different ways, "What is shattered?" and shows us in different ways that what is shattered is always our diminished view of ourselves as isolated, as separate, as inadequate, as that which so often leads us in fear to, in his words, keep "the fullness of life at bay while we negotiate our way into a safe, thin, colorless cage." Thus this work is nothing less than an invitation to liberate ourselves from the habitual and confining prisons of our own creation, to begin to listen to the inner callings and yearnings of the heart, and to literally cook in the fires of direct experience, and in doing so, to grow ripe and savory and complete in who we actually are.

The practice of mindfulness ranges far and wide and deep within the psyche and the heart. As a liberative practice, it calls us to face and honor the root causes of our individual and collective anguish and suffering, and to observe them carefully as they work on us. For one thing, it asks us to be willing to observe what actually *moves* us, the root meaning of *emotion,* and to learn to stand inside of our feelings in ways that allow us to tap their power to teach and to heal and catalyze growth, and not simply to react and be chronically overwhelmed and imprisoned. Saki breathes life into this critically important domain with extreme skill and subtlety. Daniel Goleman describes the cornerstone of emotional intelligence as awareness in the present moment, really mindfulness. Here, Saki's stories embody and explicate how an "affectionate attention," a term coined by the meditation teacher and scholar Corrado Pensa, can be cultivated and brought to feeling states, however disturbing or overwhelming, with utter honesty and self-compassion, and in this way, contribute to a profound experience of freedom and the possibility of healing wounds, both old and new.

It has been my pleasure to work closely together with Saki for the past fifteen years in the Stress Reduction Clinic. Before that, he was the first intern to come through our program. In 1979, when the clinic was born, it was inevitably identified as my baby. Now, twenty years later, it is hardly a baby and it is certainly and importantly no longer "mine." For, over the years, Saki and our other deeply dedicated instructor colleagues, under his careful and loving tutelage, have taken it as their own and assiduously honed the artistry that it relentlessly calls out of all of us. This book is ample and eloquent testament/testimony to that ownership and artistry.

We have always stressed with our instructors, which means with ourselves, that to teach in the clinic, it is essential that one teach out of one's own meditation practice, which means, ultimately, out of one's own unique being, intuition, and experience, coupled with a sensitivity for what is happening in the present moment and where things may need to go in one class or another. In this way, just as when different orchestras play the same piece of music or we visit a great poem on several occasions, no two trajectories through the eight-week program are ever the same, yet the curriculum is always the same. One can feel this virtuosity of wakefulness in virtually every word and every chapter of *Heal Thy Self.*

As this book clearly reflects, Saki is a master teacher and mentor. His courage, his vulnerability, his honesty, his passion, his intelligence all echo that mastery. As the current director of the Stress Reduction Clinic and director of all clinical and educational programs in the Center for Mindfulness in Medicine, Health Care, and Society, his work has profoundly influenced hundreds of teachers of what we now call mindfulness-based stress reduction (MBSR), a movement that has grown to more than 240 programs in medical centers and clinics worldwide at the time of writing, as well as hundreds of young physicians who trained at the University of Massachusetts Medical School. I have personally learned and grown immeasurably from working with Saki, especially in coming to understand in a deeper way the value and the sacredness of vulnerability and in learning to trust the heart's ways and its need to linger and savor key moments. His colleagues, his patients, and his students have been benefiting from his clarity, his subtle sense of humor, his keen eye, and his skill as a storyteller for years. Now the whole world will have a chance to hear within these pages this multifaceted, emotionally intelligent, supremely gentle and merciful voice in all its fullness. Listen carefully. As patient, as doctor, as health professional, as human being. It might just save your life.

Jon Kabat–Zinn, Ph.D.
Associate professor of medicine
Executive director, Center for Mindfulness in
    Medicine, Health Care, and Society
Worcester, Mass.

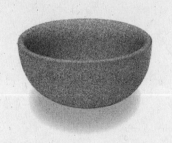

Introduction

THIS BOOK HOLDS AS ITS CENTRAL focus the healing relationship, exploring the dynamics of this archetypal connection when cradled within the practice of mindfulness meditation. It is based on the methods developed in the Stress Reduction Clinic at the University of Massachusetts Medical Center and practiced by more than 10,000 medical patients. These same methods have been tasted, firsthand, by thousands of health care professionals in training retreats across the country, often catalyzing profound shifts in their understanding of themselves, the people they care for, and the possibilities inherent in the healing relationship.

Grounded in twenty years of clinical experience, this book explores the work of mindfulness as a *Way*—an inner discipline for learning to meet and enter with awareness the challenges inherent in taking care of ourselves and serving others. Each section is an invitation—an open inquiry into the domain of mindfulness in medicine and health care. Together they offer specific methods for bringing mindfulness into your life whether you are well or facing the additional strain of illness, or you are a health care professional interested in weaving this inner discipline into the fabric of your life. I have included many chapters that might appear to have been written exclusively for caregivers or for patients. This is not the case. Rather, I have depicted a parallel, alchemical process transpiring within myself as a health care professional and within those whom I serve in the clinic when we are joined in the crucible of mindfulness. As in any worthwhile relationship, we bring out in one another exactly what is most in need of attention and what we are often most unwilling or unable to acknowledge or honor within ourselves. Our shared commitment to mindfulness offers us a powerful lens for seeing just what needs tending and a method for learning the art and craft of working with ourselves and relating to one another. As it has for the people you will meet in the pages before you, I hope that this book ignites within you a deeper understanding and trust in your own inner strength and resourcefulness as well as a keener appreciation for the unique potential embedded in the healing relationship.

Together we will explore the possibility of learning to open when we desire to close down, to face with honesty and caring attention what is unwanted and what we habitually reject in ourselves and in others, to be present to others and join with them when we wish to move away. Approached in this way, mindfulness has the potential to turn the healing relationship into an intentional sphere of lively collaboration and mutual transformation. As a way of exploring the universal, interdependent nature of this journey, I have used my own life and the lives of those whom I have encountered in our eight-week clinic course (sometimes from classes running concurrently). These stories have emerged out of the container of our shared connection. Although the names and other identifying characteristics of the people included have been changed to preserve anonymity (except in two cases where permission was granted to use the real names of Linda Putnam and Ted Cmarada), the events described are accurate and bare of affectation. For both patients and practitioners, participating in such an odyssey involves a willingness to travel like Dante or Persephone into and through the dark unknown, and only then to emerge into a previously unsuspected fullness.

In writing this book I have borrowed heavily from the thirteenth-century Sufi teacher and poet Jelaluddin Rumi. This is the food I have been raised on for a very long time. Only now am I beginning to savor and assimilate the unseen nourishment. I bow to the American poet and translator Coleman Barks for his fierce, reedlike efforts to become "an ear" and an instrument, thus making such sustenance more readily available to all of us.

Just like you, I remain a student, continually finding my way. I am bewildered and endlessly amazed by the mindlessness I encounter in myself, awed by the genius before me in the likeness of those who seek my care and give me so much, and grateful for the countless opportunities to practice wakefulness within the community of my colleagues and those whom I meet in the worlds of medicine and health care. I am extending my arm to you, hoping that, arm in arm, we can walk together for a little while into this vast, edgeless domain. Every word that I have written was spoken or shouted, sung or whispered aloud a hundred times. Take your time with these words. Whisper and sing them yourself. Say them over and over again, if you wish.

Part One

Convergence

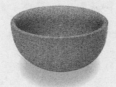

We are all substantially flawed, wounded, angry, hurt, here on Earth. But this human condition, so painful to us, and in some ways shameful—because we feel we are weak when the reality of ourselves is exposed—is made much more bearable when it is shared, face-to-face, in words that have expressive human eyes behind them.

ALICE WALKER
Anything We Love Can Be Saved

The Myth of
Chiron

LONG AGO, IN ANCIENT GREECE, the great hero god Heracles was invited to the cave of the centaur Pholos. Chiron, a wise and beneficent centaur and a great master of healing, was also present. As a token of appreciation and hospitality, Heracles brought a flask of heady wine to the gathering. The rich, fragrant liquid attracted other centaurs who, unaccustomed to wine, became drunk and then began to fight. In the ensuing melee Chiron was struck in the knee by an arrow shot by Heracles.

Then Chiron instructed Heracles in the art of treating the wound. But because the arrow had been tipped with poison from the Hydra—a many-headed monster nearly impossible to slay—the wound would never fully heal. Capable of healing others, the greatest of healers was unable to completely heal himself; and, being immortal, Chiron lives forever with this wound as the archetypal *wounded healer.*

Following his wounding, Chiron received and trained thousands of students at his cave on Mount Pelion. It is said that one of these students was Asclepius, who learned from Chiron the knowledge of plants, the power of the serpent, and the wisdom of the wounded healer. It was through the lineage of Asclepius that Hippocrates began to practice the art and science of medicine.

Living Myth

IT'S WEDNESDAY NIGHT AT six o'clock, and I'm sitting in a circle with thirty people engaged in their first class at the Stress Reduction Clinic. For the first thirty minutes we talk, skimming the surface, remaining suspended over the deep pool of a yet unspoken but nonetheless shared human experience. And then, shoulder to shoulder, we slip into this vastness.

I ask, "Perhaps you can say your name . . . something about what brings you here . . . what expectations you have . . . what you hope for, as you sit here tonight." The man on my left begins. "My name is Frank. I have colon cancer. I've had surgery . . . I've been through radiation and chemo . . . But something's not right with me. I know it. I feel it. I feel stuck, kind of numb . . . everyone in my family feels it, too. I want to live my life differently . . . with more appreciation." The class becomes still and alert as he speaks.

Everyone knows that, in his own way, Frank is speaking for all of us. The faintly audible yet unmistakable collective sigh when he stops speaking confirms this. Frank looks around, perhaps hearing and feeling as never before the reverberating impact and echo of his own words. Hopefulness brightens his eyes as he turns and looks my way. There is a silent nod between us. He closes his eyes, slides deep into the back of the chair, his cheeks wet with the tears of this pool.

Bill is on his left. He shuffles in his chair, leans forward, looks down, then begins. "My kids and I are fighting. There's tension between us a lot of the time. I really care about them. I love my work . . . it's a pressure cooker. Now I have high blood pressure. I don't like who I've become." He places his face between his hands, bends forward from the waist, and rests his elbows on his knees. His body seems momentarily enfolded in a wide, primal stillness, his eyes wrapped around years of accumulated memory. Then, drawn back into the room, he reconnects to the faces across from him and declares, "I've got to do something about it."

While Bill is speaking, the woman next to him crosses and uncrosses her legs. Right over left, left over right, unceasingly. Her head bobs up and down, matching the rhythm of her legs. Her hair falls forward across her face. She lifts it back behind her ears three or four times, then speaks in breathy, clipped bursts.

"I'm Rachel." She's quivering, trembling.

"I'm in recovery . . . I was clean." She begins to cry.

"For ten months . . . three months ago I used again . . . I've been clean three months." Now, she's sobbing.

"I've just been diagnosed HIV positive."

There's a shudder through the room. We are all sitting together, listening maybe to what our ears have never heard before—at least not at such close quarters—and do not want to hear now. I choose to console Rachel with neither words nor actions but instead to honor her truth by remaining still within the swirling water crashing against the coastline of our hearts. There is a long silence. Eyes look her way, dart my way. Closing. Opening. Silently speaking. Filling.

There are twenty-seven more stories to be with tonight. Twenty-seven more people. They know something about why they are here. Yet, as we listen together and speak, their knowing deepens. So does mine. I don't have colon cancer. I am not HIV positive, don't have high blood pressure, am not recovering from a heart attack. Yet I know that I too am addicted to a plethora of habitual emotional and mental states, sometimes obsess about my health, fight with my kids. Sometimes feel shame in the face of my perceived weakness and imperfection. Lose myself in the maelstrom of conditioned history, and know in my chest that there is really no substantive separation between them and me. For now, the present condition of our bodies is different. But behind this thin, temporary veil of demarcation, we are all patients. Patients, as captured in the Latin word *patiens,* whose root, *pati,* points to both our condition and our capacity to "undergo, endure, and bear suffering." This is our common ground, holding within itself enormous potential. If we use it wisely, it can become a seedbed, bringing forth an awakening into the fullness of our lives.

Curiously, in the midst of these unfolding stories I notice a lightness emerging. There is an unburdening here that is not simply cathartic. The most pronounced feeling in the room is not one of heaviness but one of deep acknowledgment. Such honoring is nothing less than an expression of strength and courage that feels akin to a collective rolling up of our sleeves rather than the bursting of an emotional dike that will sweep us away in helplessness and despair. It is the beginning of a relationship.

We are revealing our wounds to one another. We are naming them, but we are not being decimated by them. Quite the contrary. The usual tendency to strongly identify with and elevate "my" pain or "my" problem is slowly being dissolved in the recognition of our collective condition and in our willingness to live together, even for a few moments, inside this shared reality. There is a spontaneous arising of mindfulness—of awareness cultivated by our willingness to hear one another, to sit together without judgment, without giving advice, without reaching for easy answers or invoking shallow affirmations. Literally and figuratively we are all in our seats—perhaps more firmly than ever before—attending to and making more bearable our wounds, by sharing, as Alice Walker describes it, "face-to-face, in words that have expressive human eyes behind them."

Although I am the doctor, the teacher, sitting here and listening reminds me that I have once again been invited into a collective work. For me this is essential to remember over and over again. We will have eight weeks to explore this terrain. Eight weeks to step into an intensifying cycle of our lives ignited by our willingness to walk through the door and begin. It is not just *their* work; it is my work too. Each of us is a living myth encompassing both the woundedness of Chiron and the innate capacity to take advantage of adversity and be transformed. Beyond our roles, by virtue of being human, whether we know it or not, we are all walking the universal, mythological journey of the hero. Perhaps our real work, whether offering or seeking care, is to recognize that the healing relationship—the field upon which patient and practitioner meet—is, to use the words of the mythologist Joseph Campbell, a "self-mirroring mystery"—the embodiment of a singular human activity that raises essential questions about self, other, and what it means to *heal thy self.*

The Inner
Healer

Oh, reader ...

Whether you are in good health or ill, whether your malaise is expressed in the body or in the anguish of the mind, you have in your hands a true story. It is about a hidden treasure, a reminder of your wealth, a call to reclaim the inheritance that is yours. Do you recall the abundance I'm talking about? The gem that was placed inside you long ago. Unseen yet irresistible, it is your essence, the one walking shoulder to shoulder with you even when you imagine that you are all alone.

Can you feel this life within you? Even as you read, maybe you sense its faint stirrings in a soft wateriness flooding your mouth, or in the murmur of the old language spoken deep in your belly. You know those tones, the ones emerging from the doorway where the rib cage parts, or maybe that arise in windlike whispers filling your

13

ears in the middle of the night when sleep departs and you are summoned to wakefulness. It is your old friend, an ally that has been with you all of your life.

Maybe it's time for the two of you to be reacquainted, to travel together with fresh presence into the world. You and I are wanderers in search of this inner jewel. Despite any public relations campaigns to the contrary, despite all of our projected imagining that others have it all together, everyone is doing the same work. Maybe we can travel for a little while as companions. What other choice do we really have, anyway?

In the process called growing up, most of us have been taught to forget this innate presence. The remembering of such an inner radiance is radical. Establishing contact with such aliveness will do nothing less than turn our lives inside out. Is that such a bad deal? Meanwhile, the common conventions of the world maintain our well-oiled sense of separation, offering us thin gruel in place of real nourishment. For the most part, we remain in this fragmenting trance, until we are uprooted by circumstances that tear apart the accustomed fabric of our lives, turning us back on ourselves. Such rending is part and parcel of life. Sometimes it arrives at our doorway in the guise of illness, sometimes in the breakdown of long-standing relationships, in the loss of loved ones, in those middle-of-life eruptions that leave us little choice but to remain isolated and desperate or take the chance and slowly begin dissolving our hard, protective shells.

Fortunately, none of us escapes this reckoning. One way or another we are inextricably drawn into the deep. It is here that we begin to, as the archetypal psychologists put it, "grow down" into our lives. Here that we have the possibility of discovering within us what is most solid and sustaining while slowly learning to embody such presence in the daily round of our lives. Some would call this *Soul*. Call it what you will. Whatever it is, intuitively we know its absence and its presence in our lives. But because this reality cannot be seen, quantified, or described in our usual modes of analysis, it has been dismissed and thrown into the black box of irrationality.

This is a blind spot, a deep flaw in our cultural reasoning, that leaves us, often at the most critical moments of our lives, stripped of cultural credence and support and void of contact with a most powerful ally. Diverted by this societal bias, we turn outward, seeking this intuitively felt source of strength outside of ourselves. When staring into the face of sickness, death, the swift and decisive ending of life as usual in the face of an unexpected diagnosis, or, most commonly, when the full weight of a life half-lived begins to bear down on us relentlessly, reminding us that something is amiss, we often take refuge in outer authority, forsaking our innate strength and healing capacity.

I am not suggesting that when our health is compromised or the continuity of our physical existence is in question we abandon the advice of expert opinion and hard-won medical skill. Rather, I am saying that the power differential between patient and practitioner must be recalibrated if we are to actively reaffirm the inseparable enterprises of health care and human unfoldment. As the myth of the wounded healer suggests, there are two sides to every story. Patient and practitioner are bound together, two poles of an archetypal relationship. Remaining at the surface, we might imagine that these poles represent giver and seeker, helper and helped. But this is not the case. Conceiving it as such is too simplistic, too expedient and soul diminishing. We are each the reflection of the other. Within every health care practitioner lives the Wounded One; in every patient, every sick and suffering human being, abides a powerful Inner Healer. These are the gifts of being born into this world.

The degree to which we reclaim our reservoir of inner strength in the face of sickness, pain, or grave hardship is the degree to which, despite the gravity of the medical condition or whether we live or die, we have the opportunity to touch our undivided wholeness. Perhaps the most fundamental work of practitioner and patient lies in the recognition of the singularity of their relationship. My own experience tells me that this is so. This does not mean that the roles are the same but rather that power and the sense of limitation, irritability and excitement, fear and self-mastery, despair and compassion, sadness and joy, and all the other landmarks of healing flow in both directions.

If as patient and practitioner we are willing to revision our roles, then we have a chance to alter our relationship. In this vision lie the seeds for a new, collaborative, participatory medicine. This book is about this quest. About people who have elected, most often with the goodwill and encouragement of their physicians, to take up the practice of mindfulness and turn back toward themselves as a means of recovering their inner richness. This is my work too, and in the spirit of full participation, you will find me inside these pages. Most important, my hope is that you find yourself. As in any journey, there is risk; any deepening of character necessitates a loss. Nonetheless, initiating such a journey remains a watershed, an outpouring of unanticipated grace, an indelible opportunity to drink from the deep well of your life.

The Soft Body of
Your Calling

OH, SERVANT OF THE HEALING ARTS ...

Aren't you searching for the cure too? Aren't you curled up close, protecting that old interior soreness, that longing for remedy you secretly hope for but hardly dare to admit? Let's talk about this! How else could you possibly be of help to another? What could have drawn you to this calling if not this reference point, this open, inside wound that needs tending?

Look, my friend, we are all wounded. Welcome home! No more hiding! Fragmented and longing, aren't we all searching for the cure that will restore us to wholeness? Isn't helping simply an expression of our longing to recover this completeness? At its center, the profession of healing is the fulfillment of our wish to serve, to give—and *to be restored*. Outwardly, we direct our efforts toward restoring others, but somewhere maybe we know there really is no *other*.

Nevertheless, we hang out an attractive shingle. Perfect! Such wonder! We all need companions. Sisters and brothers of all sizes, shapes, and conditions to travel with. Wayfarers to join this caravan, to traverse this desert, walking once again toward the lush oasis, the abundant greenness of our almost forgotten lives. Why pretend that it is any different for us than for the people seeking our care? What does this accomplish? What price do we pay for this charade? Can you see that the game, the pretending itself, is a sign of something hidden and miraculous? A marvelous beguilement. An enchanting dance. A well-orchestrated seduction slowly drawing us toward some barely remembered Mystery. We are all being sought, yet we think that we are leading. Such wisdom in the ruse. Like a surprise party lovingly planned and closely concealed by those dearest to us, designed to bring us joy and contentment.

If language and music are ample evidence of a deeper silence, our wounds and flaws are sure signs of our fundamental completeness. If speech is a finger pointing toward the unspoken, our sense of incompleteness, our fragile, tender vulnerability is a sure sign of our strength. This tender softness is a portal. We hide it. Call it *flaw*, never realizing it is the entry point for marvelous possibility. Rumi reminds us of this entryway:

> *Trust your wound to a Teacher's surgery.*
> *Flies collect on a wound. They cover it,*
> *those flies of your self-protecting feelings,*
> *your love for what you think is yours.*
>
> *Let a Teacher wave away the flies*
> *and put a plaster on the wound.*
>
> *Don't turn your head. Keep looking*
> *at the bandaged place. That's where*
> *the Light enters you.*

And don't believe for a moment
that you're healing yourself.

RUMI
"Childhood Friends"

I have had my share of cuts, scars, stitches, and shots. As a child, I always looked at the needle entering the skin, the syringe-assisted movement of fluid shuttling into or out of this body, the black gut sliding through the flesh. I wanted to see. When I was little, my mother always clutched my hand and cried out, "Don't look!" And, as I got older, "Why do you look?" Fascination! As simple and mysterious as that. This is the way we fall into things. How our awareness is awakened.

Don't turn your head.
Keep looking at the bandaged place.
That's where the Light enters you.

Somewhere deep within you I suspect that you already know the truth of these three lines. Yet, despite this knowing, we are continually turning away from ourselves, from the fullness of our own experience. If we do not look at our own wounds, our own unwanted, rejected places—acknowledging, honoring, and reclaiming them within our accommodating presence—how can we possibly do this with others? During the last ten years, I have met thousands of health professionals pained by the distance they felt between themselves and those who seek their care, wishing things could be different, wondering where to begin. And I have met even more patients who have touched their own inner strength by looking into the bandaged place with new eyes. Opened eyes. Eyes willing to look unflinchingly into what is most troubling and distressing, only to simultaneously discover, in the depths, the entering light. It is here, in this commitment to awareness, that patient and practitioner can meet.

And if we keep our eyes open, we begin to discover that the healing relationship is itself a pathway, a *Way* of working with ourselves and others leading to the blurring of contrived boundaries, an awakening into our mutual, shocking brilliance, the recovery of a deep and abiding joy. For too long care has been conceived of as either practitioner-centered or patient-centered. In actuality, the healing relationship has always been a crucible for mutual transformation. The bare willingness of human beings to encounter one another in the midst of our weaknesses and strengths is the quintessential transformative agent. But my experience tells me that it is nearly impossible for us to relate to another human being in this way if we do not begin to relate to ourselves in the same manner.

To walk such a path requires a method: a disciplined way of learning to pay attention to all that is arising within. This is called *mindfulness*. But mindfulness is not simply a technique. It is an act of love. Our willingness to see, to hold ourselves closely just as we are, while being this way with another, is a revealing and deeply healing expression of care. An embodiment of compassion. Compassion begins at home, with ourselves. Whether offering or seeking help, we are all wounded and we are all whole. For the most part, we have lost sight of this interdependent actuality. Our willingness to recognize and hold such vision is an unfolding process of intimacy and healing.

The loss of normalcy, the disruption of perceived wholeness, the felt sense of isolation and limitation are at heart the primary predicament of the patient. Yet these feelings are common to all of us, whether we are caregivers or in need of healing. Helping, if it is to be healing, requires practitioners to enter into and begin to understand the disruption, uncertainty, and chaos of identity faced by those seeking their care. Because these sensibilities are a part of our commonwealth, we all have within us a polestar, a Chiron, by which to orient. Navigating in this way is possible only if caregivers learn to suspend, at least momentarily, the addictive, intoxicating drive *to do.* This requires learning how to slow down and enter—without abandoning hard-won knowledge, skill, and clinical experience—into the felt life of the patient, the person before us.

If health professionals are to help in the fullest sense of the word, then we must make this journey. This is not painless. Not the stuff of résumés. Those always suggest an ever-advancing incline, a lineage of acquisition, a smooth road of overcoming and success. No doubt there is a measure of truth in this biography. Yet if this stands alone as the standard of our unfolding calling, the vocation of becoming a True Human Being, much is lost to us and to those whom we serve.

Seen from this vantage point, those seeking our care, those we call "patients," are our *teachers*. Their instruction is subtle and deep, continually turning us back on ourselves with remarkable skill and precision. When I am willing to stop, be still, and relate directly to each situation or person before me, I have often felt, through the sheer force of their presence, the "flies" of self-protection being waved away. In so doing, a "plaster" has been applied to the wound of separation, offering instead a soothing balm of unexpected connection. In this way, we are doctor and patient for one another. Two sides of the same coin.

> *Don't turn your head.*
> *Keep looking at the bandaged place.*
> *That's where the Light enters you.*

These three lines are all the instructions we need to begin.

Part Two

Don't Turn Your Head

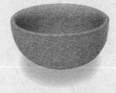

Show up.

Pay attention.

Tell the truth, without judgment or blame.

Don't be attached to outcome.

ANGELES ARRIEN
The Four-Fold Way

Week One

Our classroom shares a corridor with Pediatrics. The presence of children is pervasive. As I move out of the stairwell into the second-floor lobby, this presence makes itself known by a victorious shout of momentary escape from some unwanted insult to the body, followed by the sound of small galloping feet hotly pursued by bigger ones. By 8:50 A.M. there are ten or twelve people in the room. Shoes and boots line the hallway. Out here in the corridor, as I take off my shoes, one of the nurses just looks down the row and smiles. The nurses are used to us. Sometimes I wonder if their feet long for the same invitation, the same respite. Momentarily, we catch each other's glance, then continue on our separate ways.

In the classroom some people are talking. Some are quiet.

After a few words of introduction, I say that we will wait a little while before beginning. Then, moving around the room, I greet each person individually, shaking hands while exchanging names. By 9:00 there are more than twenty of us. By 9:05 the room is full. As I greet a woman with sunglasses sitting in the seat right next to the door, I see that she is crying. It probably took a lot for her to come through the door. Sometimes I think that getting through the door on the first day of class is the hardest thing anyone will do in the clinic. Her tremulous hand and the tears streaming from beneath her glasses attest to this.

Sitting with these thirty people feels something like waiting in an airport boarding lounge. So, as a way of beginning, I ask people to find a comfortable position and turn toward the wide expanse of windows along the western wall. Some people turn their chairs, others twist their upper torsos in the direction of the windows. Some kneel in front of their chairs, resting their arms on the seats. Many sit on the floor, using the round, colorful meditation cushions stowed under each chair. I ask them to allow their eyes to simply receive anything in their field of vision. Soon the room is silent. People become still. I suggest that we begin to notice the way the mind places names on what is seen, and whenever this occurs to simply observe it without judgment or striving while gently drawing our attention back to *seeing*. The silence accompanied by a growing stillness invites us to continue with no more words. This is our first meditation.

As this foray into attentive seeing ends, people leave the world beyond the windows and turn back toward the center of the room. Then I place three raisins in each person's hands. I don't usually do this so early in the class, but today their attention is so present and pervasive that there's no point in missing this opportunity. Using the senses of smell, touch, sight, and sound, we explore these raisins for some time. Asked simply to report their "bare" experience, people voice their perceptions with sparse precision. I ask them to try speaking in this way, simply naming, without anything extra, exactly what they are noticing. There are lots of comments. Some serious. Some funny. We go back and forth.

Our discussion feels like a cross between play and science. A native curiosity and inquisitiveness so essential to scientific inquiry is arising out of the simplicity of carefully attending to these ordinary objects. Our innate capacity for present-moment awareness is unfurling like a flag in the wind, giving rise to a keen recognition of "raisinness" usually missed in our headlong plunge into the future or our hankering for the past. Such deliberate attentiveness is, and will be, the formative ground for our work over the next two months.

Then, one by one, we slowly eat the raisins. We notice touch and taste: the subtle and dominant sensations of the body triggered by this simple act, the accompanying panoply of thoughts and feelings, the feel of pleasure and dissatisfaction. In the process the raisins move from hand-held "outside" objects to intimate "inside" elements of our bodies. Those who "hate" raisins have tried at least one. Thirty minutes into our journey, they have taken up the opportunity to work with repulsion in relationship to these raisins. They say so. Some speak openly about this, asking if they can throw the uneaten ones away. Others speak about pleasure, about wanting more, about feeling anxious when the last one "went away." We will revisit these states of mind often during the next two months.

Despite all that has already transpired this morning, we are still strangers sitting together, somewhat stiffly lining the four walls of the room. I want to be sure that we know something about where we are going, so although each person has had an individual interview explaining the details of the program before entering this room, I decide to review our itinerary. Not so much the details but the mode of travel and the commitment required. Often when doing this, I ask everyone to decide if this is where they choose to be and say that, if not, they are free to leave. Sometimes I have been taken up on this offer. Today, sitting in silence, the smiles, nods, and stillness say, "Let's go." We begin going around the room, with each person having the opportunity to speak his or her name and tell us a little or a lot about what brings them here, and what they hope for. I ask if anyone needs to go first, since going last might be hell. People laugh the embarrassed laughter of recognition; someone who says that she does need to go first begins to speak.

I could tell you about John, the surgeon who six months ago underwent open-heart surgery to repair a defective valve and who has now begun to face returning to his medical practice while trying to modify a lifetime of "habitual, workaholic behavior." Or about Dorothy, a high school music teacher with persistent angina, who says that she is always nice, never asserts herself, and feels "squeezed" most of the time. But today I'd rather tell you about Marie, the lady crying near the door. She begins her introduction with a disclaimer, telling us that the person before us isn't who she really is. Her words attest to just how much we live our lives as disclaimers—when I become, if only I were like her, when I was young, before this happened—and how easily we disown or become separated from ourselves and the actuality of our lives.

Marie tells us that what she most wants is to take back her life. She has been a high-powered businesswoman for a long time, used to being accomplished, in control, and everyone's caretaker. Now, she feels severe and almost constant anxiety accompanied by stronger episodes of terror-filled panic. She goes everywhere with a big bag—a kind of survival kit—filled with water bottles, keys, address books, an array of medicine, inspirational readings, and other items. The bag is on the floor, tucked close to her. She tells us about this bag, half-laughing, half-crying, as a tangible way of describing her predicament. Listening to her and looking her way, I wish I could see her eyes. But we have not been long enough in each other's company for me to ask this of her. I am struck most powerfully by her final testament: "I want to take back my life."

There is some silence between us, and then we have a brief conversation:

S. Can you say something about what you mean by "taking back my life"?

M. I want to be the way I was before all of this happened. I want to get back to being who I used to be.

S. Do you think that you can ever go back to who you were? I'm not sure that's possible. I'm not sure that you would want to, even if you could.

M. But I used to be so strong, so energetic, so able to handle all kinds of situations, and now look at me. I'm a mess. I've got to have this bag. I didn't drive here, someone drove me. I'm in therapy. I cry a lot—my eyes are always red. I want to get better.

S. When I said I'm not sure you can ever go back to who you were, I didn't mean that you can't, as you say, "get better" or grow, just that you have changed. You just told us that you've gone through something that has altered you. There's no telling how you will be, but if you place a memory of how you were over what you are becoming, you might close out all sorts of possibilities. Can you sense what I mean?

M. I think so.

Marie's "I think so" is filled with both relief and bewilderment. Relief born of possibility and hope, bewilderment arising out of the unsettling realization that she is indeed on a journey whose destination is no longer evident or well marked.

On this first day of class, Marie seemed to speak for many of us in the room. Each of us wants to "take back life." But what do we mean by that? How can we possibly do anything but live our own lives? Perhaps what Marie was telling us was that she wants to be more awake and alive to living her life. Maybe this was what she was saying yes to when asked if she was ready to board the plane and begin the journey. There is no telling what the outcome of saying yes will be for Marie or for the rest of us. Only time will tell. Essentially, the only thing we can do at this moment is enter into the possibility of working with the ongoing challenge invested in Angeles Arrien's invitation:

Show up.

Pay attention.

Tell the truth, without judgment or blame.

Don't be attached to outcome.

Being Present

DON'T TURN YOUR HEAD.

This single sentence conveys an essential ingredient of mindfulness practice. The words simply ask us to be present. Looking deeply into whatever is before us, looking closely at that which we'd rather not. Nothing more.

In the interdependent domains of personal health and the health care professions, mindfulness—our capacity to pay attention, moment to moment, on purpose—is an immediately accessible ally. For those in pain as well as those serving to alleviate it, such careful attentiveness is one of the most vital elements of the healing process. Health practitioners find themselves, on a daily basis, face to face with the "bandaged place." This tends to arrive in the guise of another. Yet so often it seems as if all of those whom we call patients have concealed and brought with them, into our unknowing presence, an empty mirror. Then, when we glimpse "their" torn and wounded places, we behold, quite unexpectedly, reflections of ourselves. Likewise, as patients, when confronted with illness, with the unexpected, and on the receiving end of powerful suggestions from health practitioners about our future, it is easy to turn away from ourselves, losing all sense of direction, no longer trusting our innate wisdom and navigational sensitivities.

But if, in these moments, we learn to *stop* and be present, we have a chance to learn a lot. In these moments, no matter what our role, so much seems to be at stake, so much of our identity ripe for loss, uncertainty, or displacement. And so we often turn quietly away. This is our common habit. It is understandable, because none of us wishes to be hurt. Yet because this tendency is so pervasive, our *intention,* our continually renewing vow to practice being present to the full range of our unfolding lives, is an enormous resource. My own experience suggests that the willingness to stop and be present leads to seeing and relating to circumstances and events with more clarity and directness. Out of this directness seems to emerge deeper understanding or insight into the life unfolding within and before us. Such insight allows us the possibility of choosing responses most called for by the situation rather than those reactively driven by fear, habit, or long-standing training.

By virtue of being human, each one of us is on intimate terms with *not* being present. Because of this, our intimacy with this felt absence is a powerful ally. This is the terrain of mindfulness practice. Each time that we awaken to no longer being present to ourselves or to another *is,* paradoxically, a moment of presence. If we are willing to see the whole of our lives as practice, our awareness of the moments when we are not present, coupled with our intention to awaken, brings us into the present. Given our penchant for absence, opportunities for practicing presence are abundant.

PRACTICE

Turning to the Breath

Over the course of the week, experiment with tuning in to the swing of your breath. Notice that it is possible to make contact with this ever-present rhythm in the common events of your everyday life: taking a shower, folding the laundry, washing dishes, playing with your children, writing a report, going to the doctor or seeing patients, talking with friends and colleagues, or sitting down in front of your computer are all occasions for cultivating wakefulness. Likewise, taking out the garbage, stepping into or leaving your car, eating lunch are all opportunities to stop, to see, to stay close to your life.

Turning Inside

In our modern world it has always been assumed . . . that in order to observe oneself all that is required is for a person to "look within." No one ever imagines that self-observation may be a highly disciplined skill which requires longer training than any other skill we know of . . . In contrast to this, one could very well say that the heart of the psychological disciplines of the East and the ancient Western world consists of training at self-study.

JACOB NEEDLEMAN
A Sense of the Cosmos

IN THE SERVING PROFESSIONS, the term *practice* is a generic way of describing what one does, for instance, the practice of law or medicine. Often this connotes the specific nature of people's careers as well as their relationships to the people they serve. Psychotherapists often say that they have a private "practice." Meaning: I do psychotherapy as my livelihood. Physicians speak of practice in the same manner while including under this definition reference to a particular subspecialty, such as rheumatology, family medicine, or a neurology "practice."

Curiously, almost all of our contemporary, work-defining uses of the word *practice* connote an externally directed activity done by one human being to, or on behalf of, another. Almost nowhere in our modern lexicon does the use of the word *practice* suggest that side by side with the acquired knowledge of our chosen field we are simultaneously called on to make an active, ongoing effort to work with ourselves *inwardly* if we are to engage in the full practice of our profession. Is this simply because we take as self-evident the inseparability of these twin aspects, or has something been lost in our use of the word *practice*? One of the clinic partic-ipants observed the absence of this inner dimension of practice when she said about her physician, "He's a great doctor. He knows his stuff, but his bedside manner is horrid." Health professionals may be pointing toward this same felt absence of practice when they work as hard as they can in the service of those seeking their care but find little motivation on the part of people to collaborate actively in their own health, unwilling to engage wholeheartedly in the "practice" of being a patient.

Just the other day I witnessed both this felt absence and its arrival in a discussion I was having with a group of first-year med-ical students about their initial experience of dissecting a cadaver and their anticipation about having to remove the emotion-protecting shroud covering the face of someone who, for the last several weeks in the anatomy laboratory, had largely been a leg, a thorax, an abdomen.

For the most part, they discussed the experience in clear, unwavering voices—the cool, slowly developing voices of their profession-in-training. But their comments and anticipated con-cerns about gazing into those eyes, about opening the skull, this closer encounter with death even in the guise of preserved flesh began to alter their demeanor. The flooding of associations about aging parents or grandparents, patients seen in the intensive-care unit who looked like cadavers but whose chests were still heaving and alive, or the overwhelming sense of awe and mystery evoked in their intimate confrontation with the opened body changed the tenor of their voices. Such reckoning dropped or raised the shaped breath to previously unspoken tones, made the eyes restless and wet, carried all of us into the domain of practice—turning us inward toward the barely whispered reality of our own mortality, allowing us to listen with other ears to the tremors and shock waves registering deep in the body in response to what was appearing to happen outside the personal envelope of the skin.

No one left the room that afternoon paralyzed by emotional anguish. No doubt they would head back to the lab to take up their quest. And maybe, just maybe, they would move into the vast space that accommodates the pursuit of biomedical riddles without prematurely foreclosing on the pulse and effervescent mystery of their souls. Attending closely to this revealing domain of practice would fill them out as human beings—and make them good physicians, too. No matter what our work or roles, this is the same for all of us.

PRACTICE

Meditation on the Awareness of Breathing

Meditation practice requires a disciplined, sustained effort. Yet at heart, mindfulness meditation is about care, about a willingness to come up close to our discomfort and pain without judgment, striving, manipulation, or pretense. This gentle, open, nonjudgmental approach is itself both relentless and merciful, asking of us more than we might ever have expected. To practice in such a way, awareness of the breath is an effective, ever-available means for cultivating presence.

Find a comfortable place to sit down. Sitting on the floor or sitting in a straight-backed chair is fine. If you are in a chair, see whether you can ease off the back of the chair, supporting yourself (unless you have back trouble), sitting upright yet at ease, placing your feet firmly on the floor, allowing the knees and feet to be about hip-width apart. Find a comfortable place for your hands, resting them on your lap. Try folding them together or turning the palms up or down. If you are on the floor, placing a cushion or two under your buttocks can be helpful. This will encourage your pelvis to tilt forward and your knees to touch the floor, thereby providing a strong, stable base of support. Likewise, find a comfortable place for your hands.

Now you've taken your seat.

Allow yourself to simply be with the feeling of sitting upright, solid, dignified, without pretense . . . settling into your seat, becoming aware of the flow of your breathing, sensing the rhythm of inhalation and exhalation, the feel of the breath coming into and leaving the body. Become aware of the rise and fall of the belly or the feeling of the breath at the tip of the nostrils or the sense of the whole breath coming in and going out. Rather than thinking about the breath, allow yourself to *feel* the breath—the actual physical sensations of breathing—as the breath comes in and goes out. There's no place to get to, nothing to change. Simply be aware of the breath in the body, coming and going, in and out. Each time you notice that the mind has wandered away from the awareness of breathing, gently and firmly return to the feeling of breathing, to the tide of inhalation or exhalation.

This wandering away might happen fifty times in the next five minutes. This is normal. Still, each time you notice that the mind has wandered, gently and firmly return to the feel of the breath. No need to scold yourself, no need to hold on to whatever enters the mind. Breathing. Riding the waves of inhalation and exhalation. Just this breath . . . and this breath . . . and this breath. Simply dwelling in the flow of the breath.

Coming home, returning, through the awareness of the breath, to your wholeness, your completeness. Right here, right now.

Try working with this practice for five to thirty minutes several times during the next week. If you'd like, try gradually increasing the length of time you devote to "formal" mindfulness practice.

Mirror

SITTING TO MY LEFT, he was the ninth person to speak. Poised at the edge of his chair, taking his place among the thirty of us, he told us that he was stopped by a heart attack three months ago. Forced into retirement from the construction trade at age fifty-five, he stood about five feet six inches tall and weighed about 170 pounds. Lean and strong. A great block of a man.

"My name is Chuck." His voice gained volume. "I don't know why I'm here! My wife sent me here! My doctor sent me here! My kids sent me here!"

More volume. Leaning forward, almost shouting, "And further-more, I only want to talk to the ladies in the room!"

There was a shift in the room. The men moved almost imperceptibly into the backs of their seats; in unison the women moved forward, sitting upright and very awake. With impeccable timing Chuck continued his story with ever-increasing volume. "So my wife and I were driving in town, and some guy pulled up in a car and started to give her some shit. So I got out of my car to go punch him in the face, and she yelled, 'Get back in the car.' So I came back around, and I felt about this big." (He made a small space between his thumb and index finger.) He ended with a roar: "So what's wrong if I get a little excited?"

The room was silent for what felt like eternity. Maybe ten or fifteen seconds passed, then a very brave woman on my right said, "And you don't know why you're here?" Self-conscious laughter cut through the accumulating thickness in the room, followed by an uncomfortable silence.

If the story had ended here, it might have just been a funny, ironic story. But it didn't. At that moment, with Chuck still poised on the edge of his chair—skin deep red, fists clenched, neck taut and throbbing like a plucked violin string, not laughing, just looking off into somewhere—I left my chair, slowly walked toward him, and asked, "Chuck, how long ago did this happen?" Called back from wherever he had traveled, momentarily looking my way, he raised the index finger of his right hand, inscribed a long, lazy arc for everyone to see, and said, "One year ago." Some people gasped. Most remained silent.

I could have spoken about "holding on" or about our capacity to "let go." That would have been a big mistake. Chuck said it all far more eloquently than I could. We spoke after class, and he made it clear, without any trace of rancor or criticism, that he wanted nothing to do with meditation or the Stress Reduction Clinic. Some people stood around us and listened to our conversation. Chuck spoke openly and didn't seem to mind. I sensed that looking into the mirror of his decision to drop out of the program forced everyone else to reflect on their own decision. Mirrors are like that, reflecting back to us just what is, asking nothing in return.

PRACTICE

Attending to the Quality of the Breath

As you begin to establish familiarity with the breath, try bringing attention to the *quality* of the breath when you are walking down a corridor, speaking with a colleague, patient, or doctor, when dictating notes or sitting in your yard. Note when the breath is long or short, rough, uneven, fine, light, or almost imperceptible. Paying particular attention to sensations in the body as you remain attentive to the flow and quality of the breath can teach you much. Without analysis, simply note bodily sensations such as tightness, heaviness, tiredness, lightness, pain, transparency, temperature, as you look into the mirror of your own life.

Heart

IN OUR TIME WE ARE SEEING before us in ten thousand ways the starvation and deprivation of the human heart. By *heart* I mean that part of us that feels deeply, that experiences connection beyond the confines of time, space, and linear thinking. That part of us that is moved—before thought—by beauty. That companion that aches in the loneliness of separation so often felt in our daily lives. That sweetness that longs for, and understands completely, wordless stillness and silence. That aliveness that spontaneously responds in the universal language we call *love*.

The human heart has two poles. It is an enormous, extremely sensitive receptacle—a listening device far more perceptive than the ear. And, as well, a forge of unlimited radiance, capable of converting and transmuting everything felt into warm tears, sunlight, and laughter.

For too long we have been exiled from the truth of this. The interior elders have been dismissed. The linear, discursive mind has come loose from its moorings—its proper place. We have built a boat and mistaken it for the sea. Yet behind the labels of *patient* or *practitioner*, we are all in the same boat. Thirsting for the same living water. Maybe our real work is to consciously cultivate this awakening within ourselves. If so, this work will cost us everything. It is fierce and uncompromising. Certainly this does not come by our forcing anything on anybody—including ourselves—but rather by allowing ourselves to be touched so deeply that our hearts are broken open, altering us beyond recognition.

> *The small ruby everyone wants has fallen out on*
> *the road.*
> *Some think it is east of us, others west of us.*
>
> *Some say, "among primitive earth rocks," others, "in*
> *the deep waters."*
>
> *Kabir's instinct told him it was inside, and what it*
> *was worth,*
> *and he wrapped it up carefully in his heart cloth.*

KABIR
The Kabir Book

PRACTICE

Attending to the Small Ruby

Many people more easily connect to this inner gem by remembering a being whom they care for deeply. This can be a person or an animal. Sometimes recalling an incident when someone you love was hurt or in pain can touch off waves of empathy and care. Sometimes making contact with the feeling of being cared for or

loved connects us with the life of the Heart made manifest. Deliberately recalling such incidents from time to
time might begin helping you—in the face of reason
and disbelief—to feel the truth of your own tender,
open heart. Giving yourself the opportunity to work
with this possibility is itself a reflection of your inner
ruby. What have you got to lose? What might you learn
if you simply offer yourself to this possibility?

PRACTICE

Entering into the Life of the Heart

Now and again, over the next several days, give yourself
the opportunity to pause and touch base with the "small
ruby" inside of you. You might begin to pay attention,
particularly during moments of sadness, separation, intimacy, or joy, to the texture of your "heart cloth" as
reflected in the sensations in your chest. Without judgment, allow yourself the room to feel the presence of
this inner gem. Be patient. This ruby may be protected
or momentarily obscured; nevertheless, it is adamant,
indestructible, always available.

Remember that we are learning to pay attention
without self-judgment or discursive analysis. You might
say that we are "rolling out the red carpet," welcoming—
beyond liking or disliking—whatever enters the field of
the heart. Offering ourselves such close and caring
attention is itself liberating.

Medicine
Sangha

ON THE FIRST DAY OF CLASS, after all those present had listened and spoken personally about what brought them to the clinic, I took my turn in the circle of speaking. Mostly, I do not do this, because, in the role of guide, I speak enough. Sometimes I get tired of hearing my own voice. Mostly, I want to minimize the tendency of people, particularly in a medical setting, to elevate me or to make me into the authority of their experience. Each of us must come to recognize the authorship of our own lives and to stand on the solid ground of our own experience. This is mostly solitary work.

But today is different. Today, I am moved to speak personally, intimately with these people whom I do not yet know, to voice momentarily my grief. Today, my mother is dying. She has been living and moving toward death for several weeks. She knows this and has decided to walk this unknown road intentionally.

My sister and I sat with her when she weighed her choices. She asked her doctor hard, razor's-edge questions, watched closely, and listened keenly to his responses. "How long will I have with more radiation and chemo? What will the quality of my life be? How long do I have without more treatment? What will my life be like if I don't have treatment?" This was three days ago.

In those moments her doctor sat close to her, spoke haltingly, circuitously, then straight. Struggling like the rest of us, at first resisting his own inner knowing about her impending decision, circling around again and again to the possibilities of more treatment. Asking her to explain to him, in more detail, where she stood and why, and finally . . . finally surrendering into a breathy, barely whispered "Rose, I understand." With that, my mother, sitting upright in her bed, glanced at each of us, proclaiming to herself, to the rest of us, and to the world, "I don't want any more treatment. I want to live, even for a little while, like a normal human being. To go home, to be with my family and friends, to go out and walk, to enjoy a nice meal, to go to Massachusetts once more."

Now, all of that moment, all of my slow settling into her truth, is living within me. It comes in waves, moving within, reshaping the contours of my heart. And I see that everything coming out of my mouth passes through the chest—through this pulsing actuality. This is the way it is. Since we are going to be together for the next eight weeks, and because I might have to leave class at any moment, I decide that there is a rightness in all of us knowing this, up front.

There is no melodrama in the telling. No pity in the listening. People say a lot with their eyes. Some voice their sorrow; others, their gratitude. I have no sense of breaching some taboo professional code, implicitly demanding, by my position, center stage, "disclosing" inappropriately, or implying that whatever *they* are going through pales in the light of *my* situation. On the contrary, I notice that the immediacy of life and death at the doorstep move us quickly beyond the domain of the personal into a common, universal knowing. It is palpable. There is a kind of unbearable relief. A relief born of naming rather than denying.

One powerfully built man, a security officer, drawn into this territory now revisits his reasons for being here and says a lot more. His face is flushed, beaded with sweat. He is not wearing his uniform, but if he were, it would be drenched. His gun would rust, because he, like me, is immersed in this pool of grief. A while ago he told us he was here to "reduce stress and anxiety." Now he tells us that he is caring for his mother, who is dying of cancer; that her gradually weakening condition, her episodes of intense pain, and his sense of helplessness and not knowing have become the primary source of his escalating, seemingly uncontrollable anxiety. He is in over his head, plunging downward, and in the telling discovers that he can begin to live in these dark, unknown waters.

In the ensuing silence all of us are swept into a vast, borderless place filled with dark woods, deep pools, open fields, and moonlight. It is here that our work together is being revealed. Some people speak gratefully about being able to somehow share in the living and dying of a parent. Others say they have never before spoken like this with a doctor in a health care setting. After a few minutes we move on. We eat raisins together, feel the ever-present, constantly changing breath in the belly, and begin listening closely to our bodies as we lie on the floor in the stillness of midmorning light.

Thirty strangers. Thirty different reasons for being here. Yet in our differences we are drawn together around a common intention: to learn to care for ourselves and be alive to our living; to look deeply into our own lives and to do so collectively. In this way we are actually *companions*. In the East this intentional companionship is called *sangha*. It is new to medicine.

We don't leave today having only listened to each other's stories. I gave no advice and asked others to refrain from the impulse to smooth over or attempt to immediately repair evident suffering. Instead, we have begun to learn about practice, about moving slowly yet deliberately into the world just as it is. For the next six days we won't be in class together. Each of us will be on our own, taking care of children, grandchildren, or parents, cooking, cleaning, going to work, visiting the doctor, shopping for food. Simply living our lives with the added commitment of seizing forty-five minutes of our already busy day to meditate. We call this *formal* practice. It is not easy. It is not meant to be.

In this way, we are actualizing the spirit of sangha. Each of us in our own measure is making a commitment to carry our own weight, to walk with dignity, to recognize our interdependence and yet to know that each one of us must also do this work individually. It is no one else's work. So doing, we are cultivating a firm, *internal* source of support that may, by its very nature, lend support to all of us walking this way.

My mother died during the fourth week of class. Often, I felt deeply nourished by the caring offered, mostly in silence, by the patients, as if I were their patient. We were doctoring one another, each in our own prescribed ways. Two weeks before my mother died, Lauren, a participant, gave me this poem written by Mary Oliver. It helped me.

IN BLACKWATER WOODS

Look, the trees
are turning
their own bodies
into pillars

of light,
are giving off the rich
fragrance of cinnamon
and fulfillment,

the long tapers
of cattails

are bursting and floating away over
the blue shoulders

of the ponds,
and every pond,
no matter what its
name is, is

nameless now.
Every year
everything
I have ever learned

in my lifetime
leads back to this: the fires
and the black river of loss
whose other side

is salvation,
whose meaning
none of us will ever know.
To live in this world

you must be able
to do three things:
to love what is mortal;
to hold it

against your bones knowing
your own life depends on it;
and, when the time comes to let it go,
to let it go.

I read this poem at my mother's funeral service.

Two weeks later, when I returned to class, the security officer, after offering his condolences, asked, "Do you now feel a sense of relief?" I remember him leaning forward with eyes of hope, filled with expectancy, with such desire for relief. "No, I don't feel relief." He was shattered. I was speaking the simple truth. The truth tore open his heart. He asked more questions, trying to sew together the ragged seams; then he stopped. He just nodded. I never knew what that meant. I hope he did.

Do you sense a feeling of sangha, of companionship in your life? Can you feel this body of healing? Can you sense its implications for medicine, the inherent power and simplicity of a relationship between patient and practitioner based on mutual self-inquiry, shared understanding, and collaboration? Can you imagine for yourself the deep joy and possibility of health and the healing relationship being equated with a willingness to wake up and reveal ourselves to one another no matter on which side of the relationship we sit?

Quiet Mind,
Open Heart

*The mind is the surface of the heart, the heart the depth of
the mind.*

HAZRAT INAYAT KHAN

SOMETIMES PEOPLE CONFUSE *mind* in the word *mindfulness* as
having to do with thinking about or confining attention to cog-
nition, imagining that we are being asked to engage in some form
of introspection, discursive self-analysis, or mental gymnastics.
Simply put, mindfulness is bringing a fullness of attention to
whatever is occurring, and attention is not the same as thinking.

As expressed in the quotation by the Sufi teacher Inayat Khan,
the language of many contemplative traditions suggests that the
words for "mind" and "heart" are not different. Likewise, the artist
and calligrapher Kazuaki Tanahashi describes the Japanese character for *mindfulness* as composed of two interactive figures. One
represents mind, the other, heart. Heart and mind are not imagined as separate. From this perspective Tanahashi translates mindfulness as "bringing the heart-mind to this moment."

Whether giving or receiving care, maintaining this heart-mind balance is not easy. All too often we ride the extremes—either we become lost in sympathy and the suffering of another or we find ourselves coolly observing, at a distance, aloof and uninvolved. The qualities of the quiet mind are spaciousness and clarity, the source of our capacity for discerning wisdom. The open heart is tender, warm, and flowing. Together, these attributes allow us to feel deeply and to act wisely. Even when acting means doing nothing. Perhaps compassion, in the fullest sense, is the delicate balancing of a quiet mind and an open heart. There is abundant opportunity in the healing relationship for the cultivation of such a quality of presence. But what does a quiet mind and an open heart mean? What does this actually feel like? Even though I cannot know how this feels to you, my sense is that we have all tasted this way of being. It is elusive, yet it is not something we have to get but rather something to be revealed. Something we can cultivate through paying attention. Something to be alert to, both in its presence and in its absence.

Just today, walking through the large blue fire door around the corner from the clinic, I unexpectedly encountered the shifting play of the heart-mind. I found myself face to face with a man who had been in class a year ago. I remembered him well, particularly because he had been suffering for two years with unremitting chronic back and leg pain. Because of this, he was capable of standing or walking only three or four hours a day and had young children to whom he couldn't be a father in the way he wished. He had often spoken with me of the enormous grief he felt about being unable to play freely with his kids, about his pain-induced irritability, the strain on his marriage and his sense of manhood, and the ever-present precariousness of his family's financial situation.

Given all of this, I had felt terrible when he said that he had no improvement in his pain. I remembered sitting with him during his postprogram interview, looking into his eyes, feeling both his resignation and his frustration while sensing my own slow set-tling into the truth of his experience. This happens often. Being alert to moments such as this bears enormous fruit. The desire to escape into detached clinical distance so as not to feel the suffer-ing of another and, conversely, becoming lost in one's own pathos or feeling of shame and incompleteness are equally seductive.

It was clear that both of us had hoped for more and that nei-ther of us blamed the other or felt like a failure because of his cur-rent condition. Yet we remained unsatisfied and unwilling to leave it at that. In discussing other possibilities of working with his con-dition, we had decided to set up an appointment with the Pain Clinic. When the interview ended, we walked together down the corridor and shook hands; we spoke again by telephone a few weeks later. That was the last time I had heard from him until now.

His upper torso is listing to the left, his right hand holding the wide rail secured to the wall. Shaking hands with him once again, I ask him how he is feeling. If his pain has changed. How his fam-ily is faring. He says that the pain is still big—still with him almost continually. Recent analgesic treatments have given him some relief in the back, none in the legs. He is still hardly able to walk. In his telling, I feel myself opening in response to his evident suf-fering. But my eyes are wavering—moving away from his face, from these eyes that say so much. I feel the blinking, the shifting. I suspect that to him these tiny movements are hardly discernible. To me, from the inside, they are abundantly evident, connected to the internal flood and rush of memory pulling me into the feeling of not having done enough, of wishing for more. If unno-ticed or unworked with, these waves have a way of taking over, of carving out the terrain, eroding the ground where—in this busy corridor—we momentarily stand together.

Feeling the pull enables me to stop, allows me to see that although I am standing before him, I am, in another way, leaving him all alone. Yet I am intent on not leaving. The seamless loop of the breath is an ally, the sensations in my body precision instru-ments measuring the unseen dimensions of our encounter. The willingness to attend to the transient discomfort is a small price to pay for this connection. In the midst of all this, simply returning to his eyes is enough. He is not asking for anything. Abiding here, the heart softens while the mind quiets down into a stillness and spaciousness that neither asks for nor rejects anything. Here, in the corridor, we just settle in with each other, then part when it is time.

Namaste

WHEN TRAVELING THROUGH India and other parts of the East, people greet one another with the word *Namaste*. Usually, the voicing of this sound is accompanied by a bow and the drawing together of the hands at the center of the chest in a gesture of deep respect. *Namaste* means "I acknowledge and bow to the divine in you." Each wayfarer, whether friend, family member, or stranger, is greeted in this manner. And although this gesture, like any other, can become mechanical and devoid of meaning, it is nonetheless a strikingly powerful yet simple reminder of our origins. When uttered sincerely and heard repeatedly, this reminder has a transformative effect on both the sender and the receiver. Soon enough one begins to recognize the divine in another, realizing that it is none other than that spark of divinity in oneself that is seeing and being seen by the divinity in another.

As differently as this might be embodied by each of us, I believe that the active remembrance of this reality is crucial to our lives, our work, and our well-being. There is no pretense about this. No need for elaborate theatrics, no special clothing or false piety, no funny language—just a straightforward honoring of this truth. We, and the person before us, are always more than that which appears. Something far more direct and astonishing is transpiring behind the appearances. Perhaps our real job is to sustain this remembrance in the face of overwhelming proof to the contrary. Despite the embodied evidence of stress, illness, pain, or suffering in another, and without the slightest denial of this reality, maybe our essential work is to meet another within this crucible of temporal conditions while simultaneously relating to them as nothing less than a localized embodiment of the divine. As far as I can tell, this has little to do with liking the person, nothing to do with preaching or lecturing, and far more to do with recognizing that they, like we, are simply a temporary expressions of something larger and far more encompassing.

Our willingness to relate with another in this way is fundamentally healing. Yet our culture, which has grown out of and been dominated by such a strong individually oriented ethos, continues to emphasize, rather unconsciously, the myth of domination and authority. Fueled by fear and insecurity, there is enormous disequilibrium in this worldview. When this power dynamic takes primacy in the world of caring, caregivers may begin to see themselves as the authorities—as *more than*. Held in the shadow of this point of view, patients or clients can easily begin seeing themselves as helpless, weaker—*less than*. This model is fundamentally flawed. And although the health practitioner may have knowledge and skills required by the person in need, more often than not the person seeking help has as much to offer to the helper.

Namaste! The remembrance of our collective origins. So different from "How do you do?" No question about it. Painfully uncompromising. Straight from the heart of one to another.

PRACTICE

Paying Attention to the Space Between Us

If you find yourself sometime this week sitting in the presence of a friend, family member, colleague, or patient, make a deliberate effort in these moments of shared space to attend to your breathing, to the feel and rhythm of the breath and the sensations in your body. Allow your curiosity to focus on those elements of the interaction that tend to draw you either away from or into a sense of connection. Notice the quality of the breath in each instance, allowing yourself to become curious about the nature of this personal inquiry.

See if you can pay attention to such things as the tone of your voice and the tendency to lose or to maintain the thread of the conversation depending on what's going on in your own mind and body, as well as bodily sensations such as tightness and porousness and mind states such as impatience, boredom, or curiosity. Notice if there is any connection between bodily sensations, mind states, the quality of the breath, and your actions and behaviors. Allow yourself the room to observe—without judgment—the intrapersonal dynamics occurring as the breath moves through cycles of inhalation and exhalation. Notice if there are times when you are no longer breathing freely and what is happening within and *between* the two of you in these moments. Be gentle with yourself, allowing your curiosity to be your guide.

Remembrance

BEFORE READING TO THE BOTTOM of the page and automatically turning to the next word on the next page, how about slowing down and stopping for a few moments, right now? Dwelling here, notice the weight of the book in your hands, the texture of the page, the sounds around you. Feel the swing of the breath, the life shuttling in and out of the body, the sustaining presence inside the breath. Now, if you like, speak this poem aloud, to yourself—two or three times. Try taking it slowly.

There are two kinds of intelligence: One acquired,
as a child in school memorizes facts and concepts
from books and from what the teacher says,
collecting information from the traditional sciences
as well as from the new sciences.

With such intelligence you rise in the world.
You get ranked ahead or behind others
in regard to your competence in retaining
information. You stroll with this intelligence
in and out of fields of knowledge, getting always more
marks on your preserving tablets.

There is another kind of tablet, one
already completed and preserved inside you.
A spring overflowing its springbox. A freshness
in the center of the chest. This other intelligence
does not turn yellow or stagnate. It's fluid,
and it doesn't move from outside to inside
through the conduits of plumbing-learning.

This second knowing is a fountainhead
from within you, moving out.

RUMI
"Two Kinds of Intelligence"

Now, try whispering . . . *whispering* . . . this poem to yourself as
many times as you like.

This poem is for you. Let the resonance of your own voice—
the feeling inside the voiced sounds—help you remember the
truth of your own life. Walk into where the words are pointing,
the abundance you carry within you in this very moment. Linger
here if you like, bringing attention to the breath—to the actual
feeling of the breath inside the body. There's no need to force or
manipulate the breath. No need to try to make the mind blank.
No need to get somewhere. No need to make anything happen.
Just sitting and breathing. Aware of the feeling of the breath.
Allowing thoughts to come and go without struggle, gently
returning to the breath each time the mind has wandered away

from the rhythm of inhalation and exhalation. Sitting. Breathing. Remembering.

PRACTICE

Remembrance

Sometime today, and at other times during this week, try stopping and sitting for a few moments—or a few minutes—quietly feeling the swing of the breath gliding in and out of the body. As you sit allow yourself the possibility of settling into "this other intelligence that does not turn yellow or stagnate." Take your time with this, remembering that this is not something to be acquired but something that is "already completed and preserved inside you." What will it take for you to consider this possibility?

Notice the sense of disbelief, the feel of separation, the tangle of mind waves, the aliveness of possibility and openness residing within you. Remember that neither the poem nor mindfulness practice is suggesting that you have to go about getting anything. Rather, the work is to be still long enough to touch the actuality of your inheritance.

Boundary
Making

THE USUAL MEANING OF *BOUNDARY* is "dividing line"—a separation between two things. But isn't a boundary also a place of meeting and coming together? When walking barefoot along the shoreline, are we only on the land? What about the water under our feet? Where does the land begin and end? Where exactly is the water's edge? The actuality of the shoreline reveals these seemingly solid and distinct edges as constantly in motion. They are fluid. Nonfixed. Enfolded in one another.

These intertwining movements are similar for us as patients and practitioners. Yet all too often the hard, impenetrable borders of this relationship are carved out of a process of identification that divides self and not-self into mutually exclusive entities. Unconsciously, this process winds up shaping the entire interaction. I am not suggesting that these roles are the same. They are not. But they are just that—roles. And behind these roles lies a much larger field, our shared humanness. This is all too easily and often forgotten. Yet it is the common ground of the entire relationship. Can you feel this place? How much of what we refer to as *me* is invested and confirmed into existence by maintaining these role distinctions? Do you notice how you are feeling right now, as you read these words? Can we look at this a little more closely?

Jack was a tall, forty-eight-year-old, hollow-cheeked man with AIDS. During the first day of class he shouted, "I'm so fucking angry. I'm angry that I have AIDS. I'm angry that nobody really helps me very much. I'm angry that I don't get treated very well." His rage was fierce. He shook his fists, pounded the seat of his chair, and visibly frightened some of the people sitting near him. Before I said a single word, he looked directly at me, announcing for all to hear, "I wonder if there is room for my anger in this room." In response, I simply replied that there was room here for his anger, if we were both willing to work with it over time. He nodded, sat back in his chair, and decided to stay. At that moment I didn't know what the statement "if we were both willing to work with it" really meant. I was soon to find out.

Each week Jack created a special space for himself. He would turn his chair sideways, lean his back against a wall, and stretch out his legs on two more chairs. Then he would place a clipboard and pad of paper on his lap, lift a pencil from behind his ear, and take notes, sometimes feverishly. After class he would present me with pages of questions and ask or demand that I consider them, one at a time. We discussed his questions, talked by phone about his life, and sometimes met. Jack was struggling to understand himself. He was trying to come to terms with his past, the fear and unknownness of the future, and the poignancy of the present, which found him stripped of a longtime career, money, mobility, and a sense of self-worth. Over time I began to develop a genuine feeling of warmth for Jack. Yet undeniably, when I was around him, I also felt a recurring sense of threat and accompanying contraction, whose origins I neither understood nor was able to rationalize away.

One morning at about 7:15 I took out my keys to open the door to our classroom. The door was unlocked, and Jack was already sitting in his customary place, writing. I felt instantly threatened. Meanwhile, Jack was effervescent. "Hi, Doc. I hope you don't mind that I'm here, but I got someone to open up the room for me because I've got some things to talk with you about." He got up, stepped into the wide open space created by the circle of chairs, and walked toward me with his pad in his hand. We were face to face. Only he was on one side of the chairs, and I deliberately remained on the other side.

I had drawn the boundary.

He began to talk about his meditation practice. I was scrambling, backpedaling inside. There was something so unpredictable about Jack. My mind was wild with "Why is he in my space? What does he want from me now? Why is he so damn demanding?" My speech became a series of sparse, cool utterances. I began to lose it. Contracting, tightening, and I felt sure that Jack saw and sensed all of this. But even more powerfully, I became painfully aware how, in that moment, I was actually abandoning Jack. I had hardened the boundary, retreated to seemingly solid ground, making a self-made, well-fortified barrier. I ached in the anguish of our dilemma: I feeling squeezed and impotent, he feeling isolated and unheard, each caught, at that moment, in a personally constructed reality that bound both of us in hell.

Jack's voice broke and went flat. He looked at me with eyes of bewilderment and despair. Together we stood in *confusion*—literally, *mixed together*. And, in that stammering moment of our shared predicament, something fell away. As I stood on "my side" of the chairs, I connected with Jack's eyes and then stepped into the open circle. We just stood there for a while, okay with each other. There was not a lot of talk, but when we spoke, we spoke like brothers. I was afraid that Jack wanted something from me that I couldn't possibly give him, so I had recoiled. Jack feared that I would reject and abandon him like everyone else had, so he had pressed hard and pursued. For a while we had each fulfilled our unspoken expectations of the other.

Soon after this Jack became homebound and then bedridden for progressively longer periods of time. Once when I called him, just to see how he was, he said, "Thanks for calling, Saki. No one treats me with this much decency." After our conversation ended, I remember thinking, "It was *just* a phone call. Maybe it lasted one or two minutes. So simple." I was astonished, once again, by the power and fulfillment of connection. This longing is universal.

Yet all too often it is drummed out of the heart of the professional-in-training. At the end of a combined training program for professionals and laypeople led by my colleague Jon Kabat-Zinn and me, some of the professionals were angry and said, "You treated them better than us. We wanted what you gave them." Our initial reaction was defensive. We agreed with them. We had given more to the "patients." This had been our intention from the beginning, and we had decided in advance that, as professionals, their job was to take care of themselves.

Upon deeper reflection we heard the truth of their feelings. Many of these caregivers wept over the isolation they feel and the cultural barriers of "profession" that make it nearly impossible to acknowledge these needs without feeling or appearing incompetent or weak. Then they began to speak openly about the pain associated with academic training that all too often insists on the development of a clinical distance or objectivity that had slowly seeped into the very fabric of their lives, leaving them feeling cut off and numb. For many of them now in practice, this felt like a straitjacket and caused them to wonder why they had ever endured graduate education. Each of them, in his or her own way, was experiencing the constricting and isolating nature of artificial boundaries.

Whether patient or practitioner, we are always in relationship. We are linked. Can you feel the critical need for each of us to cultivate a willingness to closely watch the *boundary-making mind* and to develop an extremely refined tool for understanding with precision this process and the distance it creates? I believe that such deliberate and careful attention is the foundation for the entire healing relationship. This begins with our individual commitment to a disciplined way of understanding the nature of mind and its effect in human interactions. Without this kind of attention, how are we ever going to create more collaborative, mutually responsive health care?

Right now, as I write, I'm struck with just how present Jack is in each word of this text. How could I have written it without him? There are no boundaries.

PRACTICE

Working with the Boundary-Making Mind

Certainly there are a distinct "me" and a distinct "you" operating in our everyday relationships with the world. Each of us comes as a unique package of qualities and conditions shaped by myriad factors. We call this "my self." Yet, when we look closely into our lives, we see that we are made up of thousands of what the Vietnamese Zen master Thich Nhat Hanh calls "non-self" elements, such things as earth, water, fire, air, space, carbon, oxygen, parents, genes from the entire planetary pool. The same constituents that make up the sun, the stars in the night sky, and the salty seas are a part of our common, embodied heritage. As the preceding story makes clear, it is easy to forget all of this in the heat of the moment.

As a means of reducing the intensity of this habit of separation, I have found it useful to be deliberate about two things. First, I try to attend to the feeling of difference and distinction when it arises within me during an encounter with another, and to bring awareness to those subtle or not-so-subtle sensations that accompany such moments. If I am awake in these moments, I attend to the feeling of the breath without attempting to suppress the impulsive desire for distinction. When I am able to work with myself in this way, I am usually in a better position to begin consciously looking for what "we" have in common. Perhaps at first it is that we are wearing blue or are about the same height. Pretty soon, the shared commonality of being human, beyond any theories or ideas about similarities, comes most tangibly into play.

In the final analysis, it is this recognition of our shared humanness operating behind our endlessly different packages that draws us back into connection. In this way it is a homecoming, a growing larger rather than a diminishment of what I think of as "me." The intention is not to wipe out the distinctions and the variety, or to compress all of us into a colorless mass. Rather, it is to discover, behind the distinctions, that we are connected and not so limited by the notion of individuality that often functions as an impenetrable barrier to belonging.

The next time the feeling of separation or distinction arises in you, try moving beyond the verbal dimension of your encounter with another. Attention to the look of their eyes, the tiny lines at the corners of the mouth, the rigidity or softness of the body, the felt sense of "their" breath, the carriage of their head and shoulders, the timbre behind the spoken word, the feelings in your solar plexus, the tone of your own voice, the feelings emanating from your own body-mind-heart, and what you say can encourage the slow dissolution of the boundary-making mind.

Week Two

THIS MORNING THE ATMOSPHERE in the room is charged
with conversation. We have not seen one another since last week;
during this week we have begun to engage together, each in our
own home, in the daily practice of mindfulness meditation. People
seem to be more comfortable with one another. Spontaneous
clusters of conversation are scattered about the space. Listening
to the sounds in the room, I hear that homework, particularly
formal meditation—a specific amount of time set aside each
day to practice mindfulness—is, in most instances, the subject of
conversation.

Agnes and John are settled in their wheelchairs. Gerry's
crutches are leaning against the north-facing windows, and Millie
has looped her cane over her chair. The vast expanse of sky
beyond the windows is cloudless and deep blue. Sitting here in this

room, we have a view of Route 9, the wide boulevard of Plantation Street, and the surrounding hills and cityscape.

At 9:05 A.M. we begin, and I ask people once again to turn toward the windows. The transition is brief as silence replaces the sound of shifting chairs and bodies. Again we practice simply "seeing." We are viewing the same scene, but much has changed in one week—both beyond the glass and inside the room. People are still, receiving, not turning so much in my direction for guidance. We sit with our eyes open for ten or twelve minutes, and in the lingering silence I introduce people to "formal" sitting meditation practice. I encourage them to stay with the silence, and after I demonstrate, both in a chair and on a cushion on the floor, the postural options for sitting meditation, we gently close our eyes, ride the waves of the breath, and simply sit.

During the past seven days, practicing the body scan meditation, people have begun to cultivate awareness while lying on their backs and systematically bringing attention to each part of their bodies. Rather than "trying" to be relaxed or enter a meditative "state," the body scan encourages the development of a more refined awareness of and intimacy with the body, which allows us to be more in touch with ourselves and our environment. Now we bring the momentum of this week of sustained practice to sitting meditation. We "sit" for fifteen minutes, directing our attention to the physical sensations of the breath as it enters and leaves the body. When we finish, I ask people to continue this practice for five to ten minutes a day over the next seven days. Then I ask if there are any questions or comments. Comments are sparse. It is 9:35, and we have been together in silence for thirty minutes. We are becoming familiar with this terrain.

Then we move to the floor and revisit the body scan. Lying here, on our backs, we practice together in silence for forty minutes. Our conversation then turns to the subject of homework. I ask people to report their experience of actually *practicing* the body scan. They have much to say. There are many comments about the difficulty of "finding" the time to practice. I remind people that

they won't "find" the time but will have to "make" it. We are facing in this first week of practice the reality of lives so full, so busy
and squeezed, that attempting to practice becomes a mirror of our
dizzying pace.

There are questions about falling asleep while practicing.
Comments about the difficulty of sustaining a regular discipline.
Observations about how much the mind wanders and is filled
with thoughts and assumptions about not "progressing" or being
"successful." Fear and confusion expressed about feeling more
rather than less pain. Anxiety provoked about the fear of becoming "too relaxed" and, therefore, "unproductive." Amazement and
awe triggered in people who report becoming aware of the
breath, both spontaneously and deliberately, in the midst of difficult everyday situations and finding it useful. Momentum begins
to build, and the pace and tempo of conversation become akin to
the feel of a strong, moving river. Simultaneously, there is a growing frankness, a less-censored willingness for people to say whatever is on their minds about the experience of practice.

Noreen is becoming acutely aware of the vulnerability of the
body while practicing the body scan. She says that she feels "much
softness in this practice coupled with waves of sadness" and recognition, on what she says feels like "a cellular level," of just how
much the body remembers and how the body scan is helping her
to embrace and care for these old wounds.

After several people have spoken, George, a short, solidly built
man, stands in the manner of a preacher and says that this week he
has tasted what it means to have "charity toward my body."
Kathleen tells all of us that she hoped that practicing the body scan
would fill her with "something," but instead of feeling full she is
feeling "empty." She is troubled by this and asks what she can do
about it. After engaging with her in a dialogue about her experience of feeling "empty," I suggest, for now, that she try living with
this feeling, allowing the feeling itself, coupled with the deepening of awareness, to slowly reveal the answer to her question. She
appears temporarily satisfied. But I am not satisfied with my

response to her. She has asked an essential question, yet at this moment more words will do little. So I sit, just like her, hoping for another opportunity, yet realizing that the right moment has already passed me by and I cannot retrieve it. For now it's better that I return to myself and to my companions, watching and listening closely.

Finally, Drew asks, "How do I reconcile wanting to accomplish something with the idea of non-doing, of not trying to get something or somewhere when I am here for a reason and I want relief?" Drew's question initiates a ripple of nodding heads like stalks of wheat in a collective response to the wind and quizzical eyes that seem to be saying, "Yes, this is my question, too!"

The sense of "stuckness" and the desire to do something about it rises like cream to the top of our discussion. Somehow all of these questions about the ups and downs of practice are expressions of a collective stuckness. The sense of entrapment is strong. Entrapments in habits, assumptions, and long-held perceptions are beginning to be seen more clearly. With the slowing down, with the being with things as they are, people are beginning to awaken to the disquieting sense of being relentlessly pushed or catapulted headlong through life. The practice itself is informing us about this reality while simultaneously offering a method to work with what is being seen. This knowing is painful. No longer turning away, we are beginning to *see* our lives just as they are. This is both revelatory and uncomfortable, the inevitable price of wakefulness.

I sense that people are now asking themselves: Do I want to participate in this program? Can I live my life in this way? What will it cost me? What am I willing to loosen my grasp on? Do I have the capacity to do so even if I want to? These are crucial, life-giving questions, unanticipated in our usual world of adulthood. Fresh and alive, they are both inviting and terrifying to everyone sitting in the room. In this moment, each of us is beginning to reckon with the challenge of "taking back my life" and the effort required to awaken to the fullness of this one life that we are living.

Right now, it feels as if each of us is standing at the edge of a deep well, staring into a shimmering unknown, wrestling with the unspoken question Do I say no to this moment, remaining parched and brittle? Or do I say yes and drink from these uncertain waters holding the possibility of a life renewed? If people decide to drop out of the course, this is when it begins to happen. As people leave today, I sense an emerging energetic sobriety. The honeymoon is waning. Like most honeymoons, it ends quickly and leaves us having to decide. We have been moved into deciding whether or not to work with ourselves in this shared community of practice. For all of us, this deciding is akin to taking a vow. We are facing a decision about commitment to a direction—to a *Way*—that is often sensed as having profound consequences in our lives.

We are each facing a turning point. One that is not manufactured by me as the instructor but is emerging out of our individual and collective willingness to look deeply into our lives via the medium of mindfulness. This is a matter of life and death. Not physical death, but the dawning realization that we have something to say about living fully or half asleep, in quiet desperation.

It is your decision as well.

Friendship

IT IS POSSIBLE THAT THE entire healing relationship is actually founded on friendship. Perhaps this sounds radical. Like most radical ideas, such as *all men are created equal ... endowed by their Creator with certain unalienable rights ... among these are life, liberty, and the pursuit of happiness,* it takes us aback at first and later begins to kindle in us a sense of possibility and freedom that is self-evident yet often given little consideration.

Understandably, we usually reserve the word *friend* for a few people in our lives with whom we feel an intimate trust. Yet when we begin to look more deeply into the feeling of friendship, what we usually mean has everything to do with endurance, understanding, a willingness to be open and assume our place in relationship to another. There is an equality about friendship that is not defined by role, knowledge, education, or status. Often what friendship means has much to do with our willingness to relate openly and directly with people and situations just as they are.

There is a strong element of loyalty in friendship. Not loyalty to country or culture but instead loyalty to the very activity of being alive. In this way, liking or not liking play little part in the actuality of friendship as it arises within the patient-practitioner relationship. Often feelings of grasping and aversion arise out of the situations in which we find ourselves with others. Certainly these varying emotional tones are grist for the mill in terms of working on ourselves, but the feelings themselves neither indicate the absence of friendship nor necessarily hinder our capacity to offer care.

Perhaps we are all seeking friendship. All wishing to relate and be related to in such a manner. Recently, I was struck by the evidence of this longing during a retreat-training for health professionals. At the conclusion of a morning of mostly silent meditation practice, we spontaneously moved into a lucid, spellbinding conversation about some of the fundamental attributes of the healing relationship. Without any prior mention or formal introduction, the quality of relatedness that we often associate with friendship bubbled to the surface.

People spoke about feeling that the nonjudging, nonstriving, generosity-oriented aspects of mindfulness practice were helping them become "friends" with themselves. As we began to explore in more depth and specificity what this felt like internally, and how this sense of friendship had expressed itself over the course of the morning, many of these two hundred participants spoke about feeling a newfound comfort with themselves no matter what kinds of thoughts or feelings arose in the mind. They spoke about a tangible lessening of constriction, a palpable sense of self-kindness, newly discovered feelings of safety, a gradual release from the endless cycles of condemnation, denial, justification, guilt, and attempted repentance.

The feeling of slowly being able to welcome—beyond liking or disliking—whatever entered the field of awareness gave people such relief, hope, and quiet embrace. The room was alive with this feeling of befriending. Spontaneously, many of these physicians, nurses, psychiatrists, psychologists, and hospital administrators began quietly speaking about the possibility of "sitting with another" just as they had been sitting with themselves all morning.

PRACTICE

Befriending Self

Mindfulness is an act of hospitality. A way of learning to treat ourselves with kindness and care that slowly begins to percolate into the deepest recesses of our being while gradually offering us the possibility of relating to others in the same manner. Working with whatever is present is enough. There is no need to condemn ourselves for not feeling loving or kind. Rather, the process simply asks us to entertain the possibility of offering hospitality to ourselves no matter what we are feeling or thinking. This has nothing to do with denial or self-justification for unkind or undesirable actions but everything to do with self-compassion when facing the rough, shadowy, difficult, or uncooked aspects of our lives.

This week try taking some time to explore the possibility of sitting with yourself as if you were your own best friend. Dwelling in the awareness of the breath, allowing thoughts and feelings to come and go, experiment with the possibility of embracing yourself as you would embrace another person dear to you and needing to be held. If you like, try silently repeating a phrase on your own behalf. You might offer yourself one or more of the following:

"May I be safe."
"May I be free from suffering."
"May I be peaceful."

Find the words that are right for you in this moment of
your life. This may feel awkward, foreign, or lacking
authenticity. None of this need be denied. Nevertheless,
if this act of intrapsychic hospitality appeals to you, give
yourself the room to work with this practice as a way of
caring for yourself. Such a way of working with ourselves is not meant to foster egocentricity or selfishness.
It is just asking us to step back into the circle of caring
and include ourselves.

Intrinsic
Well-Being

AN INTERCHANGE BETWEEN Michelangelo and a wealthy patroness of his day:

"Master, what are your ideas about sculpting?"

"Madam, there is nothing in the mind of man that is not already in the block of stone. Based on my intellect and my skill, my work is to draw forth that which is already in the stone."

It was the 1964 World's Fair in Flushing Meadows, New York. I was fifteen years old when I walked into an exhibition pavilion and saw, in all its glory, the *Pietà* surrounded by throngs of onlookers flashing cameras, kneeling in prayer, whispering softly, expressing loudly to one another the excitement and awe drawn forth from them by this figure. As moving and lifelike as it was, I remember turning away from the crowd, wandering through the hall, and finding myself standing before another of the artist's creations entitled *The Slaves*.

As I recall, across thirty-three years of memory, there stood a series of figures carved and shaped by the sculptor. To my right stood a line of adult figures, chiseled, smoothed, liberated by the master's measured strikes until the skin itself glistened and pulsed as if enlivened by his own transfused, stone-embodied life. The draped rags, following the grain and veins of stone, lay in linenlike folds. The ragged-edged garments, frayed with unerring, detailed precision, hung in captivating motion. My eyes, and so much more of me, received and became saturated by this line of carved figures. To the left of the adults stood the children. First figures well defined, then small, less-articulated faces, rag-covered bodies, standing in stillness, looking out at the world and into me across the aeons. Beckoning. Their faces marking the first blows, the rough rock, the master's original listening intention, until the final face emerged as one eye, one ear, one half-completed nose suspended in space, while the other, not revealed half remained rockbound, contained "within" the black stone that spawned this silent, motionless caravan before me.

It was one of those moments not fully understood yet somehow known. One of those moments needing slow, steady simmering over the course of years in order to be transformed into the strong, seamless bones that silently give marrow and substance to a life. One of those moments that lay coiled and alive in my deep interior, permeating, shaping, and sustaining a life, until the exchange between the woman and Michelangelo with which this story begins was handed to me by a professor of art history. After hearing me tell this tale in class, he came to the next session with the literary reference, thereby completing a circle begun more than thirty years ago.

"There is nothing in the mind of man that is not already in the block of stone."

We are all completely contained genius, being coaxed and drawn forth in a thousand ways, honed into actuality, slowly polished into fullness. This "drawing forth" is the essential education. Can you feel this action in your own life? What is being drawn forth from within you? What is being given birth?

What would it be like to approach our lives, and to engage in the lives of others, knowing we are all inherently whole, intrinsically well, in need of being drawn forth into the discovery of unabashed completeness? How would this change the entire dance of practitioner and patient? What kind of relationship would be wrought and shaped when seen from, and uncompromisingly held within, this point of view?

Shattered
But Still Whole

Seven a.m. Driving to work on the Mass Pike. Heading east. I turn on National Public Radio's *Morning Edition*. Today the journalist is in Chicago. He weaves this tale: A large, prestigious museum in Chicago raised a lot of public and private money to host an art exhibit. They chose as the theme for the exhibit the works of "disabled" artists, sent out a hundred invitations to exhibit, and received no takers.

Perplexed, anxious, and probably scared, the museum curator and board of directors, with a lot of money and reputation on the line, decide to get to the bottom of this. The answer seems obvious. They discover that none of these highly accomplished artists, many of whom have shown their work internationally, wants to exhibit under the rubric "disabled." Months later, after much persuasion and negotiation, a well-known artist who also has a "disability" consented to exhibit his work. Following this opening, other artists accepted, and the exhibit is filled.

The radio story picks up with the commentator walking through the gallery on opening day, describing to the listeners what he sees while having conversations with some of the artists. He is facing a wall-sized painting composed of extremely refined geometric patterns placed in perfect relationship to one another. He interviews the painter, asking how he does such precise and intricately detailed work. The artist responds, "This is just what I see, and I put it on canvas." The artist is blind. He has been blind since birth.

Next we hear about a sculptor. A large, powerfully built man who fabricates and welds metal, building huge and sometimes towerlike structures. We find out that this sculptor lost his leg some years ago, is unable to wear a prosthesis, and continues to sculpt with one leg. He is asked if his work now is different from when he had two legs. The man responds clearly, deliberately. "This is what I do now. This is normal." We come to find out that this sculptor has been chosen to create the centerpiece of the exhibit. He has sculpted a sphere out of stone, perhaps marble or granite. We are told that it was perfect, with an uninterrupted, smoothly polished surface. After the sphere was completed, the artist smashed it, then put it back together with bolts, metal fasteners, and bonding agents. Now—full of fractures—it is sitting in the middle of the gallery, in the middle of America, labeled SHATTERED BUT STILL WHOLE.

Hearing this, as I'm traveling at fifty-five miles an hour, shatters me. My chest is split wide open. I slow down, tears pouring out of my eyes—out of all of my fractures—cascading onto shirt, tie, and lap. Ten miles to go. Astonished! Turned inside out by tears for me, by tears for all of us. The river behind these teardrops feels immense and impersonal. These tears are not the old familiar ones that flow from tributaries of self-pity or anxiety-driven thirst for that which I don't have and desperately want. This flow is far more universal. It is a grief-bearing river. The shudder, the melting tell me in an instant that this story has pierced the tight membrane of personal history, erupting into the truth of our collective condition.

This is every person's story.

Walking through the parking lot, preparing for class, sitting quietly with the participants after listening to someone tell us about the momentous, unexpected changes in her life wrought by illness, and her recent contact with an unanticipated sense of solidity and well-being, I stand, walk slowly about the room, and tell this story. There is an immense response. People reverberate, struck like gongs by the sound—surrounded by the sound, their deep resonance with

SHATTERED BUT STILL WHOLE

SHATTERED BUT STILL WHOLE

SHATTERED BUT STILL WHOLE

With more ferocity, mercy, and compassion than ten thousand words could have conveyed, this recognition penetrates. Like mindfulness practice, the story helps everyone in the room remember that having a serious illness and being treated in a mainstream, academic medical center need not, like amnesia, numb us, nor further intoxicate us into a deep, sleepy forgetfulness of our inherent wholeness.

But too often, driven largely by time, training, and uncertainty, health professionals lose sight of or turn away from the deeper mission of engaging in the intimacy of suffering—our own, and that of those who seek our care. By necessity we have developed a vast reservoir of knowledge intended to relieve, and in some instances cure. But, like a double-edged sword, this knowledge can easily bind us to the shattered aspects of these human beings before us while simultaneously blinding us to their—and our—deeper, intrinsic wholeness. Most often this reactive conditioning arises out of fear. Fear of the unknown. Fear of the uncomfortable. Fear of helplessness. Fear of our own broken places. Yet, if we do not carefully attend to this within ourselves, we treat ourselves and the ones seeking our care unjustly. Refusing, mostly unconsciously, to acknowledge and enter into our own brokenness, we remain numb, distant, and, most often, cynical.

Yes, this river is grief bearing. And it is more. It bears gold. Just as the princess lost her golden ball in the Grimms' tale "The Frog Prince" or the boy lost his golden ball in the story "Iron John," we have all lost, for a time, our gold. As patients, having an illness creates enormous, unanticipated turbulence. As caregivers, living and working daily in the midst of the suffering and illness of others, we are each apportioned a measure of this turbulence. Because of this, we have before us the possibility of purposefully allowing all that transpires in the messiness and perplexity of the healing relationship to shake us out of our habitual ruts so that we might together, as human beings temporarily personified as "patient and practitioner," actively engage in the mutual discovery of our radiant, golden nature through the life of the relationship itself.

All of us hunger to be seen in this way. This is the source of our blossoming. It begins internally with the development of care for ourselves, no matter what our role, condition, or predicament. Later it starts to spill over and flower in our relationships with others. It is by no means a smooth road, and meditation is not snake oil, panacea, or some feel-good exercise. It is a method, a means of beginning to contact and cultivate these latent, already existent qualities. This is the true meaning of education, the essence of mindfulness—to draw forth that which already *is*—rather than imagining that we must fill others or be filled from some outside source in order to be complete. In the context of medicine, mindfulness practice, much like a sextant, offers a tool for navigating these uncharted seas whether we are helpers or ones seeking help.

Like the enfolded, interdependent actuality called "practitioner and patient," shatteredness and wholeness exist at once. Dynamic aspects contained within the larger completeness called human being. It is through the recognition and honoring of our fractures, the surface turbulence, and the deep grain of our being, that we uncover what we imagined to be unreachable. This is the root and fruit of mindfulness practice. The joining of meditation and medicine.

Part Three

Keep Looking at the Bandaged Place

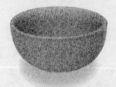

We have not even to risk the journey alone, for the heroes of all times have gone before us. The labyrinth is thoroughly known. We have only to follow the thread of the hero path, and where we had thought to find an abomination, we shall find a god. And where we sought to slay another, we shall slay ourselves. Where we had thought to travel outward, we will have come to the center of our existence. And where we had thought to be alone, we will be with all the world.

JOSEPH CAMPBELL
The Hero with a Thousand Faces

The Devil's Sooty Brother

A DISCHARGED SOLDIER HAD nothing to live on and no longer knew what to do with his life. So he went out into the forest, and after walking for a little while, he met a little man who was actually the devil himself.

"What's the matter?" the little man said to him. "You look so gloomy."

"I'm hungry and have no money," said the soldier.

"If you hire yourself out to me and will be my servant," the devil said, "you'll have enough to eat for the rest of your life. But you've got to serve me for seven years, and after that you'll be free. There's just one other thing I've got to tell you: you're not allowed to wash yourself, comb your hair, trim your beard, cut your nails or hair, or wipe your eyes."

"If that's the way it must be, let's get on with it," the soldier said, and he went away with the little man, who led him straight to hell and told him what his chores were: he was to tend the fires under the kettles in which the damned souls were sitting, sweep the house clean and carry the dirt out the door, and keep everything in order. However, he was never to peek into the kettles, or things would go badly for him.

"I understand," said the soldier. "I'll take good care of everything." So the old devil set out again on his travels, and the soldier began his duty. He put fuel on the fires, swept and carried the dirt out the door, and did everything just as he was ordered. When the old devil returned, he checked to see if everything had been done according to his instructions, nodded his approval, and went off again. Now, for the first time, the soldier took a good look around hell.

There were kettles all about, and they were boiling and bubbling with tremendous fires under each one of them. He would have given his life to know what was in them if the devil had not strictly forbidden it. Finally, he could no longer restrain himself: he lifted the lid of the first kettle a little and looked inside, only to see his old sergeant sitting there.

"Aha, you crumb!" he said. "Fancy meeting you here! You used to step on me, but now I've got you under my foot." He let the lid drop quickly, stirred the fire, and added fresh wood. After that he moved to the second kettle, lifted the lid a little, and peeked inside. There sat his lieutenant. "Aha, you crumb!" he said. "Fancy meeting you here. You used to step on me, but now I've got you under my foot." He shut the lid again and added a log to the fire to make it really good and hot for him. Now he wanted to see who was sitting in the third kettle, and it turned out to be his general. "Aha, you crumb! Fancy meeting you here! You used to step on me, but now I've got you under my foot." He got out a bellows and pumped it until the fire of hell was blazing hot under him.

And so it is that he served out his seven years in hell. He never washed, combed himself, trimmed his beard, cut his nails, or wiped his eyes. The seven years passed so quickly that he was convinced that only six months had gone by. When his time was completely up, the devil came and said, "Well, Hans, what've you been doing all this time?"

"I've tended the fires under the kettles, and I've swept and carried the dirt out the door."

"But you also peeked into the kettles. Well, you're just lucky that you added more wood to the fire; otherwise you would have forfeited your life. Now your time is up. Do you want to go back home?"

"Yes," said the soldier. "I'd like to see how my father's doing at home."

"All right, if you want to get your proper reward, you must go and fill your knapsack with the dirt you've swept up and take it home with you. And you must also go unwashed and uncombed, with long hair on your head and a long beard, with uncut nails, and with bleary eyes. And if anyone asks you where you're coming from, you've got to say, 'From hell.' And if anyone asks you who you are, you're to say, 'I'm the devil's sooty brother and my king as well.'"

The soldier said nothing. Indeed, he carried out the devil's instructions, but he was not at all satisfied with his reward. As soon as he was out in the forest again, he took the knapsack and wanted to shake it out. But when he opened it, he discovered that the dirt had turned into pure gold. "Never in my life would I have imagined that," said the soldier, who was delighted and went into the city. An innkeeper was standing in front of his inn as Hans approached, and when he caught sight of Hans, the innkeeper was terrified because the soldier looked so dreadful, even more frightening than a scarecrow. He called out to him and asked, "Where are you coming from?"

"From hell."

"Who are you?"

"The devil's sooty brother and my king as well."

The innkeeper did not want to let him inside, but when Hans showed him the gold, he went and unlatched the door himself.

Then Hans ordered the best room and insisted on the finest service. He ate and drank his fill but did not wash or comb himself as the devil instructed. Finally, he lay down to sleep, but the innkeeper could not get the knapsack out of his mind. Just the thought of it left him no peace. So he crept into the room during the night and stole it.

When Hans got up the next morning and went to pay the innkeeper before leaving, his knapsack was gone. However, he wasted no words and thought, It's not your fault that this happened, and he turned around and went straight back to hell, where he complained about his misfortune to the devil and asked for help.

"Sit down," said the devil. "I'm going to wash and comb you, trim your beard, cut your hair and nails, and wash out your eyes."

When he was finished with the soldier, he gave him a knapsack full of dirt again and said, "Go there and tell the innkeeper to give you back your gold; otherwise I'll come and fetch him, and he'll have to tend the fires in your place."

Hans went back and said to the innkeeper, "You stole my money, and if you don't give it back, you'll go to hell in my place and you'll look just as awful as I did."

The innkeeper gave him back the money and even more besides. Then he begged him to be quiet about what had happened.

Now Hans was a rich man and set out on his way home. He bought himself a pair of rough linen overalls and wandered here and there playing music, for he had learned that from the devil in hell. Once he happened to play before an old king in a certain country, and the king was so pleased that he promised Hans his oldest daughter in marriage. However, when she heard that she was to marry a commoner in white overalls, she said, "I'll go drown myself in the deepest lake before I do that." So the king gave Hans to his youngest daughter, who was willing to marry him out of love for her father. So the devil's sooty brother got the king's daughter, and when the old king died, he got the whole kingdom as well.

This tale often draws strong reactions from people who feel that "making a pact with the devil" is not an honorable enterprise by any stretch of the imagination. Often their ire is further fueled, their confusion compounded, by the seeming injustice of such a deed being so richly rewarded. Yet since the "devil" comes in such an endless variety of packages, I suspect that each of us can identify with having made some sorts of deals with the devil.

But since this story unfolds in mythological time and place, our usual ideas and opinions are not adequate to the deeper task of understanding archetypal patterns as they exist within each one of us. In order for this kind of understanding to blossom, our curiosity, our sense of not knowing, and our feeling of place within a larger unfolding universe will have to take center stage. Meanwhile, our customary sense of reason will need to recede into the wings for a time. If we allow for the possibility that all of the characters, objects, and situations in the story are aspects of our own internal architecture rather than an external set of circumstances and personalities to be taken literally, we may find ourselves becoming free enough to discover new ways of seeing and understanding.

For the soldier, life has changed. He has been discharged from a lifetime of duties and activities. Stripped of the commonplace and familiar, he no longer quite knows who he is or what is his to do. What we do know is that he wishes "to go home!" Much as in Dante's opening lines in the *Inferno,* we might find ourselves "lost" in the middle of our lives. Sometimes because of illness. Sometimes because we have come to the end of a road. Sometimes because we find ourselves at a crossroads no longer sure of which way to turn. Sometimes because the life we have lived has become depressing and unhappy and we are beginning to turn toward the uncomfortable truth of this. Sometimes because a vague uneasiness draws us inexorably toward a deeper reckoning with ourselves.

Like Dante, and like the soldier, at times we all need a Virgil, someone to lead us into the depths, into what Rumi refers to as the "bandaged place." The place we have not dared to look but which must be entered and seen clearly if we are to find ourselves anew and head "home." For the soldier, the "little man" identified as the devil becomes his guide. Up until now his life has been filled with regimen, regularity, and most probably a certain culturally derived esteem and respect befitting a soldier. But whether he likes it or not, that time has passed. Now he is homeless, cut loose from his familiar moorings. Perhaps he is strangely attracted to the unknown or has an inkling that after a lifetime of allegiance to outward duty and responsibility it is now time for him to travel, in both directions, the steep, vertical axis of his life.

He is facing the crossing of some threshold. This marks the dissolution of the identity he has believed himself to be. For all of us, particularly if we have been highly educated, groomed for success, and seen as accomplished in the eyes of the culture, this crossing begins a breaking apart of who we have imagined ourselves to be. Seen clearly and used wisely, this descent into the underworld, into the darker regions of our lives, becomes an essential part of journey home.

It is hard to know by thinking about all of this from the outside. But if we move inside, we might begin to ask more useful questions, such as Who is the soldier in me? What about the "little man?" The general, sergeant, and lieutenant—who or what do they represent? The fire, the logs, the boiling pots—where do they reside in me, in my life? Who is the one in me that relishes revenge? What aspects of myself were revealed to me in the mirror of the opened pots? What are the uncombed, unshaven, uncut hair and nails all about? The unwashed eyes? The soot? The identification of brotherhood with the rejected, unwanted aspects of my life arriving in the guise of the little man and the reward of swept dirt turned to gold? What might the old and young daughters, the marriage, the old king, and the unexpected inheritance of a kingdom be pointing at in me? What is the purpose of my life, now? What are my responsibilities to my soul?

The story is clear about this: to find our way home we must *go down*. We are asked to move underground, to examine in fine detail the unwanted aspects of ourselves. To cook, like those boiling kettles, the unowned, undesirable elements of our psyches so that, transformed, we may emerge from this purgatory capable of living our lives as songs, as new tunes. This is hard work.

The world's literature is filled with such quests. Dante's descent into the inferno; Beowulf's submergence into the lake to meet Grendel's mother. The descent into the underworld by Persephone; Ulysses' journey to the gates of Hades; Jonah's days and nights in the belly of the whale. Each of us is asked to go down into this underworld, into the darkness, to face our fears, to acknowledge and "own" all aspects of self, and in this way to be renewed.

And who is this "devil"? Do our usual conceptions of such a being include someone who gives us seven years of work? Do they include someone who asks us to remain unshaven and unwashed, and who, despite his clear warning about "not looking in the pots," forgives our transgressions and awards us with a sack full of gold—twice? Do our usual ideas of the "devil" include someone who promises us sustenance and freedom—and delivers, who acts as our intercessor when we are robbed of our worked-for rewards, washes our eyes and grooms us, teaches us to play music, and leads us into a life and livelihood that is completely unexpected and thoroughly renewing? Rather than being a personification of evil, as in some myths and tales, my sense is that this "devil" represents the shadowy, unwanted, undesirable aspects of our own lives, a source of inner guidance often rejected. Our reckoning with these forces cannot be put off forever, and our willingness to go down—to take "a good look around hell"—is necessary if we are to regain the fullness of our lives. This is a part of our universal quest, our destiny. Without a doubt disease, illness, and the worlds of medicine and health care are unforeseen entries into these darker regions.

For all of us, our willingness to explore our fears, to live inside helplessness, confusion, and uncertainty, is a powerful ally. Acknowledging our repeated exposure to human suffering—our own and others'—and the seductive draw of numbness or melancholy that provides temporary escape is necessary if we are to be renewed. Our losses, our sense of self-importance and staunch individuality, and our unacknowledged grief can all be worked with as a way of entering the deep, encountering ourselves more fully, reconnecting to our own humanity and, in turn, to the humanity of those with whom we come in contact. This is the soldier's work, and it is our work as well.

Perhaps this is why Rumi urges us to "keep looking at the bandaged place." And if we bring with us the intention to pay attention, to be aware, to feel, to no longer "turn our head away" but instead to learn from all that we taste and feel, we may enter into a relationship with the darkness that opens up all of those long-sealed, tightly held, worn-out places in us needing air and refreshment. In doing so, we might discover radiance pouring into and emanating from all of our flaws and fissures, illuminating and transforming into "gold" what has been dark and most feared.

If we refuse this journey, we may never play the music of our own lives. We might never sing the song that is only ours to sing. What a tragedy this would be. For the world needs your tune, remains incomplete without it, and waits, endlessly patient, for your voicing of your song.

Going Down

At times I felt like a thief because I heard words, saw people and places—and used it all in my writing . . . There was something deeper going on, though—the force of those encounters. I was put off guard again and again, and the result was—well, a descent into myself.

WILLIAM CARLOS WILLIAMS
The Doctor Stories

Sick *Afflicted with ill health or disease: ailing.*
Deeply affected with some distressing feeling: sick at heart.

Webster's College Dictionary

SICKNESS TAKES US DOWN, pulls the rug out from under us, disrupts the continuity. It is not pretty and, as the preceding definition points out, is not limited to the disruption of bodily functions. For all of us, this *going down* is unavoidable, ranging from the tolerable to the terrifying. Within this downward-facing world are all the small pains and discomforts we rail against, tolerate, bend to, and negotiate with in our daily lives. Included are the more catastrophic moments when the immediate continuity of our physical existence is threatened or seriously compromised, when the ones we dearly love die, and most primal, when our identity, our sense of who we are, unravels into perplexity and uncertainty.

For health professionals, living in this world of sickness and brokenness is our daily bread. Often I ask myself these questions about this world: How have I arrived here? How shall I meet this world, today? What is my job—my real job? I do not know the complete answer to any one of these questions. But like all sustained inquiry, the questing has, over time, led me again and again back to this question:

How can I allow this world to penetrate so deeply under my skin that the repeated rubbing up against those whose lives have been broken cracks me open too?

This longing to be broken open is neither masochism nor a wish martyrdom. Certainly it does not mean surrendering knowledge, skill, personal competency, or lightheartedness. But if we are to discover our capacity to engage with and accompany those with whom we work through this twisting valley, through this long calvary of the soul, then we must walk this way with them. This is not easy. Whether silently drawn or pulled roughly into this netherworld, we are always being asked to encounter ourselves when encountering the suffering and brokenness of another. Even as I write this, I sense a faint yet distinct hollowness in the belly, a subtle clenching. There is a catch in the throat because this question and its answer lie deep in the larynx:

How do we best accompany those seeking care into this realm within and below the body? The shadow region, named "distressing: sick at heart."

There is only one way. We must go there ourselves.

This going belowground is often the subject of great myths and fairy stories, as exemplified by "The Devil's Sooty Brother." As human beings and as caregivers, we are each called to this region. Entry into this domain is nothing less than a long apprenticeship. Here, we are instructed in the crafts of repetition, watchfulness, and lingering, in each moment, in each task, with each person before us, until we begin to understand, to know deep in our own bellies, that we are capable of keeping our hearts open in hell. Be forewarned! This country is, in the language of fairy tale and myth, composed of ashes, soot, and messiness. Full of the unaccustomed. The Augean stables. Here, our white coats, pressed clothes, bright smiles, appropriate affect, well-kept hair, and polished shoes are grist for soil, dark chambers, heat, and wetness.

Here, there is only one dress code: Nakedness.

As difficult as this may sound, such an odyssey offers us the possibility of recovering and cultivating our open, tender hearts. Without such labor we may remain hard and armored, "fragmented" . . . "distressed and sick of heart." And it will show. It always shows. Like a glass wall or a long shadow stretched out between ourselves and another. I am walking the same road as you. Experience tells me that our refusal to enter this Way prolongs and maintains the sense of isolation and incompleteness. Because of this we remain raw and uncooked, unaware of our own wholeness. If this was our singular fate, then this itself would be a tragedy. But this is not the case because we are not separate, independent entities. We are always in relationship, immersed in the actuality of interdependence. We have only to look deeply into how the food we eat was grown and delivered to our tables, the roots of our common linguistic inheritance, what we speak of, our longing for love, our feelings of isolation and aloneness, and our shared ecstasy with moon-filled nights, wood fires, radiant sunrises, and companionship to know that we are not separate.

This is why what happens in that alive, open space called the patient-practitioner relationship demands such close attention. It is an embodiment, a direct expression of interconnectedness and interdependence. Beyond a doubt we work on ourselves as a means of helping others and, simultaneously, working with others is a way of working on ourselves. The simple truth of this is hard to open up to because it changes the entire nature of the healing relationship from one of fixing and rescuing, or authority and domination, to one of service, collaborative creativity, and inquiry. This alone is a cracking open of our imagined sense of self and position. For our work and our privilege is to assist and accompany others into the discovery of their own intrinsic wholeness existing *behind* illness, even when death is close at hand or when one faces living with a chronic illness.

Words alone cannot convey this. What is called for, right alongside all of our medical procedures and clinical strategies, is a slowing down, a loosening of the neck tie, a rolling up of our sleeves, a willingness to leap into the breech without holding on, an intimate embracing of our own tattered hearts.

Perhaps because we are servants of the healing arts, this is our vocation and our blessing. Our degree of willingness to walk this way with another is a measure of our own brokenness and our own wholeness. They are inseparable. It is impossible to make contact with the life gushing up and out of these cracks if we are not opened. This living water is an incomparable meal.

> *Mankind owns four things*
> *That are no good at sea—*
> *Rudder, anchor, oars,*
> *And the fear of going down.*

> ANTONIO MACHADO
> *Times Alone*

The Stairwell

FINDING A PARKING SPOT near the last row of trees, I pull in and leave the car. Today's journey across the parking lot begins. High clouds, birdsong, cattails, and damp pavement are my companions. Walking and silently repeating an old Sufi koan, *"Whose feet are these? . . . Whose feet are these? . . . Whose feet are these?"* while listening for the returning, interior motions.

Almost always in this walk to the medical center, I see them resting in orderly rows, snug against the building, their chrome bones sometimes reflecting morning sun. Today, their seats hold faint whispers of wayward snow, reminding me of where I am, and where I will be for much of the day. The wheelchairs are poised between the benches, parked and readied, like welcoming sentinels, awaiting their day's work. The sign above the glass-walled lobby reads: OUTPATIENT HOSPITAL ENTRANCE.

Stepping into a glass wedge of the circulating door, momentarily looking out into the sprawling lobby, I am swiftly delivered to the tiled entryway. Silently ushered into this open area, I encounter three people: an elderly gentleman clothed in green cap and matching work clothes limping with a cane; a middle-aged woman draped in a big tan coat and bright yellow sweater sitting in a wheelchair; an adolescent boy, leather-jacketed, with severely twisted limbs, walking with great courage and great difficulty across the lobby. This is all revealed within the first thirty feet of entry. There is more. And, when I allow myself to see, to really see, there is always more.

Every workday for the last fourteen years I have entered the hospital at ground level and then *descended*. The clinic is in the basement. To get there, I must step into the stairwell. Like all wells, it takes me down. Descending today, I have companions. They are going as fast as they can. To match their rhythm, I am forced to slow my pace. From this slowing arises seeing. Down the stairs, in front of me, I glimpse exhaustion and overextended effort in the face of a thirty-five-year-old man, who, I guess, is heading for the Pain Clinic. His gait, the stiffness of the left side, the delicacy with which he meets each stair, reveal this. Not far behind him is an elderly man, with well-worn, white-knuckled fingers clutching the handrail, moving slowly, deliberately, one step at a time, accompanied by his caring, watchful wife.

Sliding my hand along the rail, I grasp momentarily the place he held, silently seeking something of him suspended in the painted steel pipe. Reaching the bottom, we pass over the threshold, catching brief over-the-shoulder glimpses of one another while holding open the blue steel door. There is a big black *A* on the door. A Level. We have arrived. If these first few minutes on the job are not enough of a reminder to me about evanescence, fragility, and my own sure destiny, I am further reminded. There is one stainless steel, Plexiglas-sided crib parked in the corridor. The IV pole and electrical monitoring unit attached. No occupant today. Sometimes the cribs are full. Images of my children dance in the mind and vanish.

The mythical symbolism and deep meaning of "going down"—of going "underground"—does not escape me. But, like all symbols, these only point a finger at something much larger and far more direct. Here, in this place, there is no need for symbols. Here, concepts turn easily into a resistance to what actually is. In this place, whether you go up or down, you will see the same thing. Here, there is sickness and suffering. It is evident everywhere. For me to do my job, it is unavoidable and necessary to remember and face this daily. When I do not, the consequences are grave; I find no place to stand, no place to be connected.

In this way the practice of "hospital mindfulness" is not different from the practice of some Buddhist monks in Southeast Asia journeying to the charnel fields for nightly meditation. I have been told that each night they choose a different body to contemplate. Sitting with the bloated body, the burned body, the partially decomposed body, until over time they are able to open fully to death, to the fear of suffering and mortality, and to learn to face this with an open heart. Perhaps they are learning to accommodate suffering and not be blown away. To embrace it gently, while recognizing and steadfastly dwelling in a larger reality that includes the entire scope of what it means to be a human being.

Sometimes, I am blown away.

This is the practice: To experience the creeping numbness, the momentary refusals, the sense of helplessness, the feel of remaining open. In this willingness I am continually discovering the deep seeds of life in this basement. As in all good wells, there is water here. It is from here that life begins. This is the wellspring of practice. It is from here, from this place, that everyday "hospital practice" gushes. Make no mistake about it, this practicing is nothing less than long retreat. Walking down the corridor to my office, I am full. Full of a strange and grateful joy. Buoyant and secure in my assignment to this oasis.

Week Three

CLASS IS FULL BY 9:05. Everyone is dressed for yoga. People wear sweatpants, sneakers, baggy clothes. I'm wearing a tie. Ferris, my dear friend and colleague, sees me just before class and says, "Saki, you're in a tie. It's yoga! Are you going to do a Clark Kent?"

"Yes, I'm going to do a Clark Kent."

During the week, three people decided to drop out of the course. I spoke with each of them. One man was in too much pain to drive forty-five minutes each way. The other two, a man and a woman, said that they didn't have the time for such an intense commitment. Both said that the intensity and demands of "this type of program" were not for them.

We begin by sitting together—no windows. Just sitting. Afterward, we slip our shoes back on, prepare to go to another room, leave books and bags behind, and take up our mats. Some people need two or three to be comfortable; there're plenty to go around. And, just before we leave, I talk about the *how* of finding our way to the largest open space in the medical center to practice yoga together. Since we've been lying down, eating, sitting, talking, and being silent—the basic elements of being alive—it's now time to practice walking. Giggles abound in the knowing truth, the punctuated reality of just what we are doing together in this medical center. This seemingly paradoxical low-tech medicine we are engaging in.

So today, before yoga, we learn mindful walking. Demonstrating in the classroom, I clear up any misconceptions about walking like zombies, about being somber or acting pious. Then I make clear to everyone the path we will follow and the availability of wheelchairs, assure Arlene that her three-wheeled scooter is a perfect vehicle for practicing "rolling" meditation, and remind those who walk particularly slowly, for whatever reason, that they need no longer rush, feel left behind or subjugated by the sense of not going fast enough because we're all going to walk s l o w l y. Not contrived. Not Chaplinesque. Not "truckin" like R. Crumb characters. No imitations of *Night of the Living Dead*—just slow, mindful walking.

Mats in hand we leave. Some people step into the elevators, others go down the stairwell; we merge in the front lobby of the Joseph Benedict Building and begin. In the gathering silence, some passersby just stare. A few smile. As amply evidenced by their rolling eyes, some wonder to themselves, others say aloud, "Goin' campin'!" Thirty adults silently walking across the campus on this May morning, greeted by the dominating green, the floating fair-weather clouds of this early New England spring. The grass is dewy, glistening, lush, the white sidewalks arrayed with green-stained etchings of grass-covered lawn mower tires accented by running borders of newly turned flower beds and freshly raised hillocks encircling the trees.

How unusual for there to be silence! My classmates are engaged, attentive, alert. In this way we are helping one another.

A few people whisper, hoping, no doubt, to break the embarrassing silence, the uncomfortable unfamiliarity. Mary and Jim form the vanguard, proceeding with cane and crutches, given permission by what we are doing together to walk as they usually do— this time with less distinction and difference. They have traveling companions. Some people slow their pace even more, making sure that Jim and Mary remain a connected part of our migrating band. Entering the medical school, we pass through the lobby now doubling as an art gallery, abundant with large, brightly colored canvases. Then we make our way east and arrive at the Faculty Conference Room. Usually home to medical lectures, slide presentations, research seminars, luncheons, today it is home to yoga.

Large drapes cover the wide expanse of windows and sliding glass doors; opening them lets in sunny, courtyard-contained light. People begin to take off their shoes, unroll and stretch out their mats, and find comfortable places to lie down on their backs while I create a walking lane for those unable to practice the yoga today, or for those who wish to move out of the yoga at points along the way. Mary will sit in a chair, and together we'll adapt the postures and turn them into "chair yoga." Cane in hand, Jim has already begun to practice walking meditation along one wall of the room. Arlene has parked her scooter beside her mat; gripping the handlebars, she leverages herself onto the floor with a well-honed smoothness that reveals just how often she has repeated this movement.

There are eight floors of hospital beds, laboratories, pharmacies, surgical suites, intensive-care units above us. Many of the people now lying stretched out on these mats have been occupants of these regions. But today, we are all alive, walking, rolling, moving, choosing to enter more deeply into relationship with our bodies no matter what our particular medical history. I am once again amazed by the willingness of people to suspend judgment, explore their bodies, put aside all the media misnomers about yoga, and simply lie down on the floor and encounter themselves directly.

For more than an hour we've practiced yoga, laughed together, and been silent while gently and purposefully working the edges, the present limits of our bodies. We've listened closely to the messages arising from deep inside this envelope, felt some of the usual boundaries give way while allowing others to remain. Our final posture is mat rolling. People meet this task with as much care and attention as any other position. We roll them tightly, tie or secure them with Velcro straps, and sit together on the floor for a little while discussing how it went. Then we slip on shoes and head back to our regular classroom.

Although we walk the same route, it is no longer the same Way. The silence has deepened; the steps are less contrived and awkward. Faces are softer, opened out more fully to the world. Some people are walking in the grass. Back in the room we begin to discuss in more detail the yoga as well as the previous week's homework. The discussion goes deep very quickly. For the most part, people have enjoyed the stretching and sustained effort, amazed that something so gentle can be so substantial. The conversation moves quickly toward the difficulty of practicing at home this past week. Comments run the gamut and include hating or loving the body scan, finding it refreshing or quite difficult to sit alone for fifteen minutes, feeling both frustration and wonder at the incessant restlessness of the wandering mind, and wanting to be but not always feeling relaxed, calm, or self-disciplined. Some people speak about the "feel" of previously undetected exhaustion, about beginning to taste a sense of quiet, applying what they are learning during formal practice as a means of handling everyday stressful situations differently, and falling asleep each time they practice the body scan.

It is obvious that we are all beginning to cook. We are learning something more about ourselves than simply being relaxed. There is enthusiasm, but it is slowly being tempered by the friction of our intentions meeting the reality of our lives when contained within the crucible of a sharpening awareness. All of us are sensing what we are actually up to, here, in this second-floor classroom, and in our lives, as we prepare to leave today. There is the definite ring and reverberation of a more sober tone in these last thirty minutes of class. Not somber. Not futile. Definitely sober.

Like moths encircling a candle flame—attracted, seduced, fascinated by something known yet never completely defined or pinpointed by the thinking mind—we are, each in our own way, being drawn into something deeper and more alluring than we could have possibly predicted three weeks ago. We are being inextricably drawn back into the circle of our own lives. The last half hour of class was no less than a collective shudder, an encounter with the true nature of our work, the first signs of the Thaw. An entrapping, long-encrusted numbness is slowly splintering and giving way. We are yielding to our depths, descending through these cracking, opening places into the deeper watercourse of our almost forgotten lives. The door opens. The room is filled with the signs and scents of melting. People walk away moist and dripping. No one is turning their head.

Digging Deeply
into Our Lives

KEEP LOOKING AT THE BANDAGED PLACE.

In the domain of mindfulness practice, taking up the invitation to not turn our heads ushers us quite naturally into "the bandaged place." For both practitioners and patients, our willingness to enter the moment-to-moment actuality of our lives takes us into this darker, unfamiliar region. By virtue of being alive, each of us winds up willingly or involuntarily traversing this terrain time and time again. Without doing so, we would remain sad and incomplete, living a life devoid of deep and abiding joy. For the most part, this is solitary work. Nothing less than our own labor is required. Yet in the midst of this journey, our family, friends, and some of our close colleagues have much to offer us by way of their honesty, support, and understanding as we walk into these little-known regions. Although no one else can do this work for us, the cultivation of community committed to mindfulness practice can sometimes be quite useful.

Rumi refers to our crossing over into the bandaged place as "the work of demolishing." Listening to his poem of guidance entitled "The Pick-Axe," see if you can allow it to touch within yourself the harsh, compassionate, resonant ring of truth living inside the words. Try reading it aloud; let the power of your own voice and what is ignited by this voicing do the digging.

Some commentary on I was a hidden treasure,
and I desired to be known: *tear down*

this house. A hundred thousand new houses
can be built from the transparent yellow carnelian

buried beneath it, and the only way to get to that
is to do the work of demolishing and then

digging under the foundations. With that value
in hand all the new construction will be done

without effort. And anyway, sooner or later this house
will fall on its own. The jewel treasure will be

uncovered, but it won't be yours then. The buried
wealth is your pay for doing the demolition,

the pick and shovel work. If you wait and just
let it happen, you'll bite your hand and say,

"I didn't do as I knew I should have." This
is a rented house. You don't own the deed.

You have a lease, and you've set up a little shop,
where you barely make a living sewing patches

on torn clothing. Yet only a few feet underneath
are two veins, pure red and bright gold carnelian.

Quick! Take the pick-axe and pry the foundation.
You've got to quit this seamstress work.

What does the patch-sewing mean you ask. Eating
and drinking. The heavy cloak of the body

is always getting torn. You patch it with food,
and other restless ego-satisfactions. Rip up

one board from the shop floor and look into
the basement. You'll see two glints in the dirt.

Rather than simply being satisfied with an analytical reckoning with our dark, unwanted places—what Jung referred to as the "shadow"—this poem suggests that within each of us, behind the purview of discursive analysis and psychological insight, lies a "hidden treasure." This "jewel treasure," these "glints in the dirt" are ours to mine if we consciously do the work of "prying the foundation."

In our own Western literary traditions, fairy tales and myths are filled with references to "gold" arising unexpectedly out of internal, subterranean labor. Engaging in such a labor inevitably leads us into a series of little deaths. Not death in the physical demise of the body, but nonetheless a death of much of what we have imagined ourselves to be. Thus, we are led into a deeper discovery of who and what we actually are.

The work of reowning our own shadow is essential. Without undergoing this labor we remain blind, unconsciously driven by these unattended-to forces. For all of us, this work is not pleasant, but it is necessary. Here we are faced with the enormity of our greed, ignorance, shame, grief, and humiliation. Looking into the mirror, we see, without filter, our capacity for deceit, self-deception, and false grandeur. We begin to fall. And through this fall, we are given the opportunity to reunite all the fragmented, seemingly disparate elements of our lives, discovering that we all carry within us, each in our own measure, the faces of everyone and everything—horrific and beautiful—that we have ever loathed, denied, dismissed, or rejected.

In this way we are slowly broken open, and we are humbled. Yet through this very same process it is possible that we will begin to enter into our wholeness as the veils of separation and self-grasping that have been so seductively drawn closed for so long are peeled away. Confronted in such a manner with ourselves, with what we have imagined to be our "self," allows us to loosen our grip on our deeply held addiction to separation and specialness. As a consequence, our capacity to feel connected to life, in all its myriad forms, begins to ripen as we arise like the mythical phoenix from the bed of our own ashes.

It is possible to go about such work consciously. I have discovered time and again that when I am willing to be present to what I encounter inside the patient-practitioner relationship, what is occurring at home in my family life, and in my interactions with colleagues, these all become sources of guidance slowly cooking me into fullness. This "look into the basement" does not require that our lives fall completely apart. Sometimes a harsh and decisive fall does occur—maybe through unexpected illness, a divorce, the death of a loved one, or being summarily fired from a job and asked to clear out of the office in fifteen minutes. But it need not be this way. There is a middle path. Perhaps we don't ask for the fall, but when it arrives we commit ourselves to attending to it purposefully. We use it like the wind to clear us out, or like a sail to fill us or set us onto another course or life trajectory. Of course, we are never fully in control of any of this. It simply consoles us when we say such a thing.

Recently, a physician with a highly regarded subspecialty who has been in practice for more than twenty-five years said to me, "I came into medicine as a king; now I'm a pawn." He is not alone in his feeling. Yet, rather than denying the truth of his predicament or succumbing to frank cynicism, he is using this feeling to understand himself, his relationships, his limitations, and his practice of medicine. In short, he is using this "fall" from the throne to feed himself and grow in unexpected ways. Some of the machismo attached to his subspecialty that has soaked and stained his skin over thirty years of training and medical practice is fading. He is a good doctor, and his native color is returning.

There is "a hidden treasure" in all of us "desiring to be known." The path leading to the discovery of such a treasure carries us invariably into and through "the bandaged place." Our inevitable entry into this place cannot be bypassed forever. No doubt something will be lost along the way. Yet our fears, uncertainty, insecurity, helplessness, intuition, and longing for authenticity and brightness are themselves nothing less than guidance along the way. Given our individual and collective predicament, we have little left to lose . . . and much to be discovered.

PRACTICE

Awareness of Thoughts and Feelings

Rather than imagining that all the moments of feeling closed down, fearful, or distant are "sins" to be confessed or repented for, explore the possibility of allowing your sense of curiosity and inquisitiveness to blossom out of these clear moments of awareness. The heart-mind is a vast, fenceless field, full of the unexpected. Often, where we hope to find joy we discover grief, where we expect pain we discover gold. Give yourself plenty of room to roam freely in this field. The rules are different here. When was the last time you were invited to play without the pressure of winning or losing breathing down your back? Give yourself the space to look around and learn. Traveling with the breath and with the intention to look directly and lucidly at what is—without preference or judgment—diminishes the feeling of a soap opera and gives rise to a straightforward, compassionate knowing.

Taking your seat, sitting upright and at ease, become aware of the breath. Give yourself the space to enter into the breath, slowly allowing the breath to come to its own rhythm. Aware of bodily sensations, the swing of the breath, the sounds around you, allow the breath to take center stage. Let your awareness of the breath deepen. Notice sounds arising, thoughts arising, emotions arising and passing without the need for censorship. No need to reject any of this. No need to view any of this as a distraction from the awareness of the breath. Simply allowing whatever enters the field of awareness to be lightly touched and let go.

No need to hold on to anything. No need to push anything away. No need to censor the mind. Rather, dwelling in the awareness of the breath . . . in this moment, and this moment. Simply sitting with awareness of the breath. Not needing to manipulate anything. Not needing to get anywhere. Simply aware of sensations arising and passing away. Allowing awareness to touch, to penetrate to the deeper levels of sensation without manipulation.

Allowing the field of awareness to expand so as to become aware of the arising of thoughts. Noticing that, anchored in the awareness of the breath, you can include in awareness these bubbles and cascading waves of the mind coming forth and passing . . . everything held within the nonstriving envelope of the breath. No need to analyze the content, rather becoming curiously aware of the process, the motion of thoughts, emotions, sounds coming and going, moment by moment. Not needing to grasp. Not needing to push away. Simply aware of moment-to-moment change. Aware of the oscillation, the ebb and flow, the flux we usually identify with as "me."

Sitting. Aware. Noticing the relationship between arising and passing away, the coming and going arising of itself. Moment-to-moment flux. Thoughts coming and going, events arising and passing within the open spaciousness of the mind.

The Woman
Beside the Well

THERE IS AN OLD CELTIC TALE about the five sons of the Irish king Eochaid. As the story goes, the sons were out hunting and got lost. Unable to find a way out of the wood, they became increasingly thirsty. Then, one by one, each of them went off seeking water. Fergus was the first of the sons to go. After some time he spotted a well and made his way to it, only to find an old woman guarding the source of refreshment. Joseph Campbell, in his book *The Hero with a Thousand Faces,* describes this woman:

> Blacker than coal every joint and segment of her was, from crown to ground; comparable to a wild horse's tail the grey wiry mass of hair that pierced her scalp's upper surface; with her sickle of a greenish looking tusk that was in her head, and curled till it touched her ear, she

could lop the verdant branch of an oak in full bearing;
blackened and smoke-bleared eyes she had; nose awry,
wide-nostrilled; a wrinkled and freckled belly, variously
unwholesome; warped crooked shins, garnished with
massive ankles and a pair of capacious shovels; knotty
knees she had and livid nails.

Standing before her, Fergus only commented, "That's the way
it is, is it?" The horrific lady responded, "That's the very way." He
then asked her if she was indeed guarding the well. "I am" was all
she said. He, in turn, asked if he might take away some water, and
she obliged him. But first, there was an agreement to be made. To
receive the water—the sustenance of the well—Fergus was
required to kiss her. He refused outright, vowing in the strongest
of terms that he would rather die of thirst than give the lady a kiss,
and he turned away. One after another, three more brothers followed the same path as Fergus. Each found the well. Each refused
to kiss the woman standing guard. Each vowed to die rather than
to make contact with the hideous presence before him. Each
turned away.

Finally, the fifth brother, the one called Niall, took up the
quest. He found the well, met the lady, and upon hearing the
terms of the bargain, agreed without hesitation not only to kiss
her but also to embrace her. When he had willingly done so, right
before his eyes the guardian of the well transformed from a distorted figure to a beautiful woman. As the story goes, Niall, daz-
zled beyond belief, described the woman before him as "a galaxy
of charms." To which her only reply was, "That is true indeed."
When asked who she was, she revealed herself: "King of Tara! I am
Royal Rule."

Standing in her fullness and true nature, she bid Niall take his
water and go back to his brothers. Before he departed, she
bestowed on him a blessing for himself and his children, that they
should be graced with the kingdom and the highest of power.
The great lady went on to say that although Niall first saw her

as ugly and distorted, he, unlike his brothers, was guided by his deep and gentle heart, offering her loving-kindness rather than revulsion. This alone, she proclaimed, is the "royal rule": To meet the unwanted with kindness and love rather than harsh rejection or abuse.

As we begin our journey into "the bandaged place," this story offers us much guidance. It asks us to see what is before us. To make deep contact with the unwanted, opening our hearts at our own pace and proceeding with gentleness rather than with the intention to deny, reject, or destroy. As the story suggests, proceeding in any other manner will keep us thirsty, held fast by concepts and ideas, views and opinions, unable to step out into a larger domain of being. There is much grief and sadness connected with living our lives in such a manner. Take note. The other brothers were not cursed, demeaned, or punished for their unwillingness to "kiss" the unwanted. Instead, they simply remained thirsty. Parched. Hard and dry. Unwilling to embrace the guardian of the well, to face, join, and work with the unwanted within themselves, they received no sustenance.

There is more than enough water for all of us. The story suggests to us a way to proceed, a way to enter, without self-loathing or paralyzing fear, into the bandaged place. At first, entering the realm of our broken or unwanted places is terrifying. Later on, we may begin to discover, through our willingness to proceed with care, an inexhaustible source of life.

PRACTICE

Learning to Embrace the Unwanted

Every day there are hundreds of unwanted moments arising like waves from the undifferentiated sea of our lives. Over the course of the next two weeks, attempt to begin working deliberately with this frothy wetness guised in the arrival of the unwished-for. What might happen if, even for a few seconds, we ceased the frantic activity, the denial, self-recrimination, or rejection usually accompanying such moments? See if you can live for a few moments or minutes with things exactly as they are. Notice sensations roiling within your body while allowing yourself to attend to conditioned gesture patterns as they manifest, or the torrent of thoughts and emotions cascading forth when you are confronted face to face with the undesired. Allowing all of this to be a source of information rather than another occasion for self-criticism is, much like the attitude and actions of Niall in the story, receiving and embracing the unwanted. When you commit yourself to cultivating such an inner stance, there's no telling what might happen.

Separation and Longing

WE HUMAN BEINGS LIVE inside such a tight cocoon. Because we are not so different, I know, whether you say so or not, that you and I live most of our lives in this stifling, unsatisfying, airtight encampment. We have named this self-woven world "I." "Me." "Mine." Frantically running from the Mystery of who or what we are behind all the extras of title, status, and role, we have reified and made special this cocoon world, making it small and solid, calling it "self." In our time this process has reached its zenith. We are in a dark enclosure. Can any of us say with absolute honesty and certainty that we are content with this state of affairs?

Tragically, while we continue weaving this secure blindness, our world has reached its nadir. Separation is the way of the world. This is true for all of us. From this mistaken identity spring greed, strident individuality, and the destruction of planetary community.

I cannot easily assign meaning to any of this. Rather, I have come to feel the truth of the situation while gradually learning to take responsibility for it. We are at a cusp, a turning point in history. We can go on living in this hard darkness, pretending that it does not exist, feeling helpless and cynical because we know it does, or we can begin to peer into this darkness, allowing the eyes to adjust, seeing with gradual clarity that which is before us.

Rumi's opening section of the Mathnawi, "The Song of the Reed," begins: "Oh hear the reed flute, how it does complain and how it tells of separation's pain . . ."

Rumi tells us that the pain of separation, the longing of the reed pulled from its source, is both a lament and a fiery, triumphant call to return—a remembering of our fundamental inseparability. Yet our experience of separation is unavoidable and holds within itself the metamorphic energies of transformation. It is our willingness to make contact with the experience of separation that allows us to touch and reckon with the full force of our longing for connection. It is the intensity of this longing—literally our willingness to live intimately with the discomfort and anguish of separation—that is the threshold and pathway leading through separation to joining.

Longing is not often spoken about in our Western psychological traditions. Desire is discussed, but desire and longing differ. Perhaps desire is the surface and longing the depth of our wish to belong, feel secure, at home. Often I sense that desire is territorial, concerned with furnishing the cocoon, making it secure, well-fortified, special. Longing in the fullest sense feels far more like the pull to move beyond the cocoon, to enter a larger stream. Longing is an enormous, barely tapped force in our lives, a tremendous pull toward a substance that we are starving for but that gets revealed at the surface level of consciousness through our culture's attention to soap operas, romance novels, and sexual enticement. Most often this energy is used to sell cars, televisions, bedroom sets, and, sadly so, ourselves—a mass seduction full of momentary heat and little light. We are hungry for intimacy, for a sense of belonging buried deeply in our being. For patients and practitioners, mindfully taking our place within the healing relationship is both an expression and a Way of embodying this innate impulse.

I often sense that, more than desiring cure, people long to belong. I know this within myself and have witnessed it hundreds of times with others. I am sure you have, too. Certainly all of us want relief from pain and physical illness, but the relief of suffering, even if there is little change in physical pain, is a healing balm, a transformation beyond expectation. Most often when this occurs it is because we touch something deeper and more fundamental within ourselves. We feel connected, whole, filled with an undeniable sense of belonging, no matter what the condition of the body.

Our privilege and responsibility as servants of the healing arts is to create an environment, provide a method, and inspire people to touch what we, beyond any evidence to the contrary, know is who they really are because we have touched this within ourselves. When people drink even a single drop from this well, longing and intensity are once again awakened, allowing the work of coming into one's fullness to be reignited. The healing relationship, when grounded in mindfulness practice, provides a bountiful laboratory for this possibility.

Week Four

TURNING AGAIN TOWARD THE WINDOWS, we sit in silence. Eyes opened, simply *seeing,* allowing these magnificent orbs to receive whatever enters the field of vision while attending now and again to the breath, to the sounds around and within us, but mostly to life touching us as seeing. Then, without break, moving into closed-eyed silence, entering the internal landscape, and after some time, back to open-eyed receiving of what the day offers to us at this moment. Thirty-five minutes of silence. During this time, someone in the corner becomes restless, begins to cry, shifts places, then picks up bag and shoes to leave. I whisper as she passes me, "Are you leaving?" Wet cheeked, she nods. "I'll come with you." Standing in front of the elevators, she's upset, angry, frustrated, and says she is having a strong reaction to the scents and smells in the room. She doesn't want to leave but can't stay in this environment.

"Damn it! I've asked people not to wear perfume or cologne."

"Yes, damn it," she echoes.

We agree on a strategy, and decide to open the door and find her another chair so that, sitting half in and half out of the room, in the cool air of the open corridor, she might be able to stay. She's game! The open door allows the usually muffled sounds of the Pediatrics Clinic to be received in vivid proximity. Cries, wails, laughter, soft sobs, small-voiced, inaudible dialogue between kids and adults filter into the room. The click and slide of heels moving across the tile, the clink of metal crutches, the high-pitched ring of elevator buzzers, nurses conversing in the hallway, the pervasive telephone, all received in our silent, still-bodied exposure to the world passing outside of our usually concealed space. Surprising sounds greet the ears: "Look, Mama!"

"Shhh!"

After a little while, the door slams shut. She's gone. A passing wave of anger, swiftly changing to sadness, then momentary futility arises, and I resolve to call her later. The smell that sent her away is still here! And as I move around the room, I find myself sniffing like a hound, seeking out the trail, looking for the source. I try to be discreet, wondering if anyone notices, thinking to myself, "I'm crazy." I find no origin.

We didn't have time enough for discussion last week, and I want to know more about what is happening for people in terms of practice. How hard or easy they may be finding it to actually practice. If and how what they are learning is beginning to percolate into their lives. What is difficult. What they are discovering. But I also want to make the space so that they can tell one another, because although we practice together in class, for the most part we have been practicing at home, on our own. This is essential and it is difficult, particularly in the early stages. The time is right for this discussion. Our individual and collective capacity to observe, to see and feel our lives more clearly, is developing. It is essential for us to have the opportunity to discuss this openly.

Tina, a slight woman with long-standing, chronic fibromyalgic pain, begins. In the early weeks of the course she found it hard to practice but now says that she is practicing more regularly. She says that she feels as if she is facing a wall. That actually there are walls on all sides of her and that she is beginning to feel just how much of her life she has cut off and "become numb to" in the process of trying to wall off and distract herself from her pain. She goes on to say that she is beginning to realize that there is a direct relationship between physical and mental pain, and that in her attempts to cope with her constant, uncomfortable physical condition, she has also cut herself off from her emotions and from the wellsprings of her life. Her speech is slow and deliberate, reflecting an openness to her predicament not previously revealed. She says that she's beginning to feel the entrapped compression of her nose, shoulders, and back against these walls and knows that she has created these tight boundaries as a way of feeling safe and secure. Now, she sees that she is in a prison of her own making.

People are nodding affirmation and recognition. Together, we are beginning to acknowledge and open to the ways in which, over time, that which provides us safety and security so often becomes our cage. Ellen shapes and articulates for all of us the cutting edge of this awakening. "I've known all of this for a long time, but *being with it* is a lot harder than just knowing it."

I recall attending a party some twenty-five years ago and becoming aware of the caged talk, the deliberate evasion of depth, the painful avoidance of anything of substance evidenced by the clutched glasses in hand, the well-placed, blinding masks of directed smoke, the ambience of lifeless pleasantry reflected in darting, lightless eyes. I too was a protecting, painfully knowing participant and accomplice. At some point, an hour or so into this deadly ritual, within the tight confines of the kitchen, a friend of mine, without agenda, uttered something so personal, so honest and direct in our huddled conversation that the entire party went silent. It was as if we'd all been waiting, scanning the airwaves like radio receivers, secretly hoping for such reception. How else could we have all heard his sounds at the same time?

When speech returned to the speechless, the entire atmosphere was altered. People began to sit on the floor, take off their shoes, hunker down in the corners, settle in to the possibility of being with one another. Actually, of being in the company of one another's attentive, listening ears and truth-telling tongues, as the night stretched out before us in the touching, spell-broken amazement and simplicity of community.

And so it is today. In this room, after three weeks of deep foundation-digging work, the work Robert Bly calls "bucket work" and Rumi names "the pick and shovel work," people begin to peel back the disguises and face the images reflected in the mirror of sustained practice. Today, Tina began this for all of us. She has run her leg, passing the baton to another. Without self-condemnation, psychological babble, melodrama, or pretense, people speak of having been asleep, stirring from a dream, feeling cold and long caged in numbing, protective hardness. There is anger about this. And more so, there is deep grief in the recognition. It has arrived unexpectedly, without invitation. Yet there is little evidence of rejection or helplessness. People are learning to see clearly, and simultaneously to hold what is seen in a caring, curious, witnessing embrace. Nonetheless, this is not easy work. The repeated force of these encounters is palpable, present, now undeniably borne within the resolve of individual commitment and the shared compact of community enterprise.

All of a sudden, in the middle of all of this, my eyes receive simultaneously two round objects hanging high up on opposite walls. "What are those things? They weren't here yesterday." And as I ask, I know! Someone, no doubt with good intentions, has placed two air-freshening units in our classroom. They are what drove Cecile away. Standing on a chair, I pull them off the walls and throw them away. As time passes, the air begins to clear, and we continue. Esther says she is crying a lot, she doesn't know why. Sometimes it happens when she is feeling quite peaceful, sometimes in unpredictable situations. In the past three classes when she has spoken about her life, she has remained suspended in the past. But today is different. She is painting us a picture of her past to help inform us about her present, and this is where she stays. She does not know why she is crying or why she is willing to accept this as a part of her life "after tiring of and then refusing to cry for years." Yet she is not trying to figure it out! She says that for now she is willing to give herself room without needing to know why.

Likewise, David says he is shocked by the vividness of the world, stunned by the tears streaming down his cheeks at the traffic light or the kitchen table, and wonders just how much he has missed and what has remained for so long unseen. Gina, much like Tina, is taken aback by what she is beginning to learn about herself. She begins speaking about a creeping hardness that has found its way into her life, shaping her reality and her responses. She is dumbfounded, bewildered about where the years have gone and where she has been all of this time. Jack, recovering from prostate cancer, says he's never been so relaxed. Philip is amazed that he is feeling "better" even though his back pain hasn't changed. He doesn't know what to make of it.

Conversation is long and lively. People express frustration with their lack of decisiveness, their procrastination, or their recognition of long-standing habits and patterns being stirred up and illuminated in the stark, simple directness of this thing called practice. They are beginning to see that the boredom, tiredness, restlessness, busyness, fear, and desire for distraction and escape that are arriving daily during formal meditation practice are none other than the far too familiar states of mind arising in their everyday lives. This makes for intriguing fascination rather than overwhelming debilitation. An openhanded curiosity and attraction are developing. People are beginning to contact a deep longing to know themselves and to direct that knowing toward the living of their lives no matter what their medical condition. No matter what has brought them into this room. Soon we end. The room is buzzing with conversation. No one wants to leave. Like our lives, our work this week lies before us. We are ignited. Looking into the "bandaged place." Ready to proceed!

But it is not quite over.

Out in the hall, on my way out of the rest room, Carla, a tall woman in her early sixties, stops me and says she'd like to have a telephone conversation with me this week; she doesn't say why. We arrange to talk the next day. We had a zesty exchange in class this morning. Perhaps I was too blunt. I knew she was uncomfortable, but I refused to relate to her as other than the powerful adult that she is, even though she often recedes into a childlike whimper that, by her own admission, holds beneath it "enormous rage." The forcefulness of the encounter was my way of reminding her who she really is. It was deliberate. I know that she can stand on her own feet in a brief, stiff wind. She does too!

The next day I learn that she's angry with me about an incident that occurred three weeks ago and has now decided to talk with me about it. Although something I said about a scientific study had nothing to do with her, at least as far as I could tell, having no prior knowledge of the meaning of that event in her life, she informs me that I was "pushing her buttons." That I was "unnecessarily zeroing in" on her by speaking publicly about people in her age range, even though my comments were positive and supportive of elders and the plasticity of the human body when slowly, deliberately, and patiently engaged, over time, in regular exercise.

And so we discuss this, then talk about yesterday, which also angered her. She has thrown me back on myself, asking me to examine more closely my own actions, to look more intently at my motivation, self-righteousness, and arrogance. This is not particularly comfortable. So what! She is asking of me only what I have asked of her. She is relating to me as I choose to relate to her and, most important, the way she is learning to relate to herself.

How extraordinary that we can do this for each other. I have the distinct feeling that we are, like the rest of the participants, beginning to stand together, shoulder to shoulder, each doing the required work in our own way. I apologize for any hurt I may have caused her. She responds by saying clearly and directly, "Now I feel better." After a few moments of silence, she speaks with new authority. "Saki, I want you to know that my mask is slipping. I'm finding it difficult to always be nice, to say the right thing, to be pleasant and congenial all of the time the way I'm used to. I know that this is right, and it's terrifying."

Such knowing. Such strength and conviction in the voice of this woman. I am intoxicated and sobered by the power of the human spirit expressed in Carla's commitment to living. As our conversation comes to an end she thanks me, stands firm, once more clarifying her position, saying she is appreciative for being seen and spoken with as an adult. We say good-bye, understanding one another a little bit better.

By this time in the process, class never really ends. The location simply shifts. Everything encountered through the lens of mindfulness is now seen as none other than meditation, none other than life itself. All of us are listening closely and entering into our lives in a new way, reflecting in our lives, and in our commitment to living, the words of Mary Oliver in her poem "The Journey":

> . . . *and there was a new voice,*
> *which you slowly*
> *recognized as your own,*
> *that kept you company*
> *as you strode deeper and deeper*
> *into the world,*
> *determined to do*
> *the only thing you could do—*
> *determined to save*
> *the only life you could save.*

A Labor of
Love

MUCH LIKE THE CAREFUL POLISHING of a mirror, mindfulness asks of us a steady, deliberate paying of attention to our lives moment by moment. Our intention to slowly begin to polish the mirror of the heart is a fundamental activity of being a human being, not different from flossing our teeth, washing our faces, or putting on our clothes. Meditation is central to this polishing, and sustained practice is no less than the taking up of a catalytic path of development—a constantly renewed decision not to turn our heads but to learn to see and work with whatever appears before us.

The process of opening what has been closed, of touching what has been untouched, of feeling the actuality of what is, is a difficult labor. The words of Thich Nhat Hanh, the Vietnamese

Zen master and poet nominated for the Nobel Peace Prize, point
to this process:

> *Mindfulness is revealing and it is healing.*

The "revealing" is healing, functioning like a doorway, offering us
the possibility of entering a place where we can begin to understand firsthand, perhaps for the first time, the actual feel, contour,
and breadth of our lives. If wakefulness is our inheritance, our
capacity for mindless activity is a highly refined, intergenera-
tionally acquired skill. Much like the first four brothers who met
the woman at the well, we are often on automatic, out of touch
with the truth of our experience. Given this, the extraordinary
range of anguish we are faced with on a daily basis provides further impetus to shut down, become numb, function on autopilot,
aware only at the outermost edges of awareness of the immensity
of human suffering—including our own.

Whether we are offering or seeking care, our inability, for lack
of a sustained inner education, or our unwillingness to slow down,
to look deeply into our bodies, minds, and hearts has powerful
consequences. Mindfulness is inviting us to do just the opposite.
Rather than shutting down, mindfulness is inviting us to face the
immensity of suffering, including the shutting down, on purpose.
Walking this way, we are offered an opportunity and a method
for stepping into this forge. In our willingness to examine the grief,
separation, and distance we feel in ourselves, and in our relationship
to others, we open ourselves to the possibility of transformation.

The cultivation of self-knowledge shaped and made adamant
in the crucible of silence, stillness, and community is the basis of
mindfulness in medicine and health care. Our willingness to begin
with ourselves, embracing the fullness of our lives, whatever the
landscape, is where practice begins. When such a practice becomes
the core of the healing relationship, we encourage the same willingness in others. This is necessary if healing is to occur.

By healing I mean our willingness to feel and hold in awareness all parts of ourselves without division and distinction.
Essentially, this is the embodiment of self-generosity and appreciation, an expression of our fundamental wholeness, no matter
what our condition or situation. For ourselves and those with
whom we are privileged to work, this is deeply nourishing.
Receiving such sustenance has much to do with *non-doing,* with
not seeking or trying to do something or get somewhere, but
instead with learning to stop, to take our seat no matter how
painful or uncomfortable. Approaching our lives in such a manner
is a labor of love, an opportunity for each of us to give birth to the
presence of our true nature. Like any worthwhile labor, this is not
painless, but it is filled with the possibility of joy, ease, and new life.

PRACTICE

Cradling the Heart

As the "revealing" dimension of mindfulness practice
unfolds, we might begin to sense a rawness of heart, a
feeling of tenderness, vulnerability, and spaciousness
quite unfamiliar and seemingly unbearable. This feeling
is part and parcel of an open heart. Much of what we
bring to these moments is colored by thinking, imagining that what we are facing is impossible to handle or
that we are unworthy and unlovable. Working with all
of this, it is possible to move into and through the turbulence of the mind to the discovery of a wordless,
empty, openness of heart.

In the following meditation I am using the chest as
a focus of attention, but of course if we looked inside
the physical chest, we would never find this knowing
organ we call Heart. Nonetheless, our language is filled
with references to this domain of life and to its existence
in the chest region of the body. What all of these refer-

ences are pointing toward may be no less than a matter of life and death for each of us.

You can explore this meditation either sitting or lying on your back, with your legs outstretched and uncrossed and your arms comfortably alongside your body. If you are lying on the floor, placing a pad or blanket underneath you can be helpful. If you need a small pillow under your head, feel free to use one.

Having found a comfortable position, bring your attention to the breath, allowing yourself some time to settle into the flow of breathing. If you like, bring attention to the body as you lie or sit here, to the sensations of warmth and coolness, ease and agitation, lightness and heaviness, solidity and transparency . . . the feeling of contact with the floor, chair, or cushion, the awareness of sounds, inside or around you, noticing the passing play of thoughts and emotions . . . lying or sitting here aware of the breath . . . aware of the teeming life of the body . . . the feeling of holding yourself upright or of being supported by the floor. Being breathed . . . supported and held within the outstretched arms of the breath . . . not needing to do anything or to make anything happen . . . living inside the flow of the breath, the awareness of life presenting itself as sound, as thinking, as emotion . . .

Now, as you feel ready, bring your attention to the center of the chest, becoming aware of whatever sensations arise from this region . . . aware of the chest . . . of the feeling center called the Heart. Feel the swing of the breath, the movement of inhalation and exhalation, allowing the motion of the breath to become like the slow, steady motion of a cradle. Gently cradling in awareness your tender, open heart. Rocking . . . cradling . . . holding the heart with care and kindness . . .

cradling . . . gently moving . . . allowing the safety, the embrace of the breath and the cradle of support to nourish you . . . allowing you the security and the space to get to know yourself . . . to become familiar with your warmth and tenderness. Breathing . . . rocking . . . cradling for as long as you like . . . for as long as you need . . . Allowing the healing dimension of mindfulness to be revealed in the discovery of your open heart . . . in the heart willing to accommodate everything without rejection or judgment. Breathing . . . aware . . . open to the vastness of the heart . . . the grace of this moment . . . the grace of simply being yourself. Rocking . . . breathing . . . cradled in the warm embrace of your heart.

Fear

I GOT A CALL FROM Barbara on Tuesday. I hadn't seen her in about a year. When I arrived her mother was sitting by her side like a battered, world-weary, steadfast sentinel. An old lioness, relentlessly guarding the fragility and integrity of her daughter.

Barbara lay stretched out on the bed, bandaged across the belly, visibly uncomfortable, attempting to raise her energy into a barely audible hello. She was exhausted and weak. There was fear in her eyes, but something else stood out far more clearly. Her spirit, that gleam of determination that I'd come to know in her, in the face of overwhelming medical odds, had faded. In that moment, I knew that she knew this too, and that this was what had initiated her phone call and brought me to her bedside.

As we spoke together, her mother took the Road of Invincibility. Inserting, every few seconds—right in the middle of

Barbara's uncompromising description of her condition—what a beautiful daughter she had and how she was going to beat this, bounce back, and be well. And that they were going to do this together. Meanwhile, Barbara was walking, with heavy steps, the Road of Naked Truth, reporting in bare-bones, present-moment detail the condition of her body, the poor prognosis, her love for her doctor and her perceived sense of *his* helplessness, and the physical pain she was experiencing. Like a pedestrian, looking to the right and left, I stood at the intersection listening to both of them, feeling my way into the traffic.

Then Barbara told me that she had listened to my guided meditation tape before surgery, had the surgical team rewind and continually play it during her operation, and woke up to the sound of my voice in the recovery room. She was so appreciative, and so much an embodiment right there in that hospital bed, of all that she had accessed within herself during the clinic classes and throughout her long illness. Not just because she was using the tape but because of her presence while standing in the strong wind of all that was happening in her life. I felt admiration, awe, and pride.

Her mother was silent during this recounting, simply nodding her head in agreement now and again. Barbara went on speaking, returning to her prognosis. She said that because she had taken massive doses of steroids during the last ten years, the doctors had told her that it was likely her sutures would not hold because her "insides were like butter," and they weren't sure where to go in terms of her medical care.

"My insides are like butter."

Something behind those words gripped me in that moment. My own insides felt like butter too. Nausea, revulsion, and a strong desire to get away arrived with enormous force. I cannot say for sure what it was, but something about what she said activated strong fear within me. As she continued to speak, I was conscious of moving out, fading away, no longer being present. Stepping backwards down the Road of Invisibility, I eventually escaped her room. Slinking down the corridor, stepping alone into the welcoming asylum of the stairwell, I felt ashamed, utterly unsatisfied, momentarily relieved.

Even as I write this passage, I notice the strong desire to go on, to tell you about my next encounter with Barbara. To redeem myself in your eyes—and in my own. What will you think of me? What conclusions will you draw about me from this tale? How can I prove to you that I am a kind, genuine man, a competent caregiver? This is poison. More separation. Living within the swirling vortex of these voices, it is clear to me that the unwillingness to acknowledge this truth is far more destructive than the fact itself. My defendedness is more pushing away, more denial. Do you hear that this is more than personal "confession"? This is our collective work as human beings. We were not taught this in school.

The curriculum is always before us. Right under our noses. Can you smell it?

PRACTICE

Working with Fear 1

When we begin to look closely into our lives, we soon discover that fear is ubiquitous. Our usual habit when feeling fear is to protect ourselves, through either suppression or separation. As that encounter with Barbara portrays, it is easy to get caught in this reactive cycle. Feeling fear is not the issue. In many instances fear is a healthy response to a situation. Our work has far more to do with knowing when we are fearful, the ways that fear typically shapes our thoughts and actions, and the slow learning that it is possible to work *with* fear rather than either deny its existence or be driven by our conditioned intensity when fear arrives.

During the week, make it a point to begin noticing the tiny shock waves of fear that color much of your life. Notice that it is possible to stop, attend to, and feel the fear while remaining aware of the breath, and that this can be quite helpful. Rather than using the breath to "sweep away" the fear or to wage war against the bodily feelings registering on your internal Richter scale, see if you can gradually soften, allowing yourself to be with the waves of feeling just as they are. Getting acquainted with fear is all that is being asked. How much time you wish to spend inside these moments is up to you.

.   PRACTICE

Working with Fear 2

When we encounter new situations, it is not unusual for us to feel fear as well as a subtle sense of fascination or the desire to look more closely. But because of its intensity, fear usually minimizes our awareness of and movement toward curiosity.

As you begin to establish a sense of self-trust through your willingness to turn toward feelings of fear, you may start to notice that oftentimes standing right beside fear are curiosity and a sense of mystery. In almost all instances the arising of fear signals our arrival into new territory. Life is beginning to enlarge around us, and we have an opportunity to step into rather than away from it. Try working with this possibility, seeing if you can sense a nondiscursive, investigative fascination percolating through your experience. When you catch the scent of this presence, see if you can orient yourself toward this quality of attraction without needing to deny any feelings of fear. Notice if attention to this domain silently draws you into further discovery.

PRACTICE

Working with Fear 3

As you become more familiar with the terrain of fear, see if you can begin to work with the possibility of *surrender*. Allow yourself to open more and more to the feeling itself and to the possibility that you have within you the capacity to let down your guard and give yourself over to the moment. Your capacity to allow for such a moment is mindfulness itself. Your view of who you are, what fear is, and how you stand in relation to it may slowly be altered forever.

Groundlessness

WE ARE ALL SEEKING solid ground. Yet if we look closely we see there is really no such place to stand. At first, feeling this is frightening. So we spend almost every waking moment constructing stability, devising borders and boundaries in an attempt to define and solidify our turf. How exhausting and unsatisfying. This is particularly evident when we are faced with a life-altering event, a medical emergency, an unanticipated diagnosis, a crisis in the lives of our children. It is in these moments that our usual sense of turf is undermined. Often this is the requisite condition for entry to the clinic.

People arrive feeling insecure, uncomfortable with the changes in their lives yet wanting to do something about all this. They often say they feel shocked, enraged, discouraged, depressed, weighed down by helplessness and confusion. Yet all of these ingredients are the sparks and kindling for transformation. People come in a state of turbulence—what physicists call perturbed. This perturbation is groundlessness itself. The splintering of the stable, the counted-on, the taken-for-granted, the known. Because of this, these moments may also be catalysts for deep, unanticipated development. Often this is the spot where the work of mindfulness begins, and as you can see in the unfolding process of the weekly classes, people with medical conditions ranging from life-threatening to chronically uncomfortable begin learning how to dance with uncertainty, using it as a ground for the discovery of previously unforeseen possibility.

Likewise, to enter fully into this place with another asks of us as health professionals a comfort with being in this space with ourselves. Literally, a willingness to step into open, unbounded space one moment after the next, dancing at the edge of chaos while catching the tendency to stray, to revert to old habits, to fill in the empty spaces. To do something. Anything! Yet helping informed by mindfulness often means *not* doing that which is expected or desired. To do this well, nothing must be promised, save the promise of uncertainty, the open field of possibility.

PRACTICE

Working with Uncertainty

Perhaps there is no such thing as solid ground. Perhaps much of life is lost in trying to carve out such a fictitious place. In the hundreds of moments throughout the day, the week, the next year, give yourself the room to begin exploring this notion of solidity. Notice how much of your time is spent trying to construct a sense of permanence. Begin to pay attention to the myriad moments outside or within the healing relationship that you try to construct and fortify a known, inviolate world. Does this create more or less tension, more or less hardness, more or less joy? Notice what takes place in the body and the nature of the waves that crowd the mind when you grasp for such a place. Experiment in the living laboratory of your life with what might happen if you spent less time constructing an imagined state of stability and learned instead to ride the waves of your life.

Perhaps for all of us there is a treasure waiting to be found within the vast net of our lives usually referred to as uncertainty!

Riding the Green Line

I WAS LIVING IN BOSTON and had begun to see clients privately. The Green Line passed through my neighborhood. Back then the cars were ragged and run-down. Funky. The closest thing Boston had to a trolley. In the depth of winter those trains, traveling sometimes above, sometimes belowground, were sweltering. The heat was uncontrollable, nearly unbearable at times. To ease the airless, intoxicating effect, we rode that day with the windows wide open. The snow was falling as we made our way through sometimes white, mostly dirty streets, down Huntington Avenue into Jamaica Plain, surrounded by the sights and sounds of kids playing along the tracks, pelting their passing targets.

Streetcar filled to brimming. I was standing, clutching the overhead pole, swaying to the mesmerizing music, the hazy glow of self-satisfaction. In my mind, thinking about—actually congratulating myself for—the fine work I had just done with a client, bathed in how good that felt. How good I was. Remembering also, in passing, the difficulties with another, my worries about him, coming to the conclusion that "he" must be "resisting." Wondering what I was going to do about him. Wondering how I was going to make things better; then swiftly squirming away from the intimation of helplessness, the fear of incompetency.

Quickly turning from thoughts about him back to me . . . How good I felt to be helping, to be needed. Then, in that very thought-moment, smashed in the face through an open window by an ice ball. It passed through the eye of the needle, missing the people sitting by the window and those standing in the aisle so close to me. Stunned, embarrassed, and bleeding, I turned my eyes toward the floor, momentarily held by a gleaming, gray stone planted in the center of that sphere delivered with precision by the arm of the Unknown.

Deciding. Actually, *deciding* suggests too much conscious intent; knowing by being shaken, shown by having my face literally rubbed in it, "No more clients until you get to the bottom of this needing to help, this needing to be needed."

The shadow of helplessness, the fear of helplessness is partner to "helping." Keep your eyes open. Look for it. It will teach you much. I am its student.

Helplessness

I HAVE NOTICED WITHIN myself that helplessness sometimes comes clothed in a guise of helping that easily carries me into doing, planning, frantically scurrying about, imposing concepts on self and others. Born of fear and self-dissatisfaction, it is a trap and a subtle form of manipulation. Have you ever noticed this within yourself?

Much of the time this behavior is unconscious, escaping our everyday awareness. Yet, curiously, it is also deliberate. This is a strange and painful paradox. Because the truth of this paradox is so hard to take, we refute and reject it. In so doing we deceive ourselves. Even worse, we do violence to our tender, vulnerable hearts. Unable to hold lightly the intensity of not knowing, of not having all the answers, all the solutions; unable to hold the fragility of helping, of this human activity fraught with ambiguity, with loss, with endless twists and turns, we do what is most natural, most culturally credible. We refuse this vulnerability. Unwilling or unable to sit inside the tension, we take action.

Personally revisiting these mind states and openly discussing them with my colleagues has revealed that in most instances the source of this refusal is uncertainty. Uncertainty about ourselves. Uncertainty about what our job is and is not. Uncertainty about how we will be perceived. Uncertainty about the validity of our own existence. So we try hard to fill this embarrassing, uneasy uncertainty with action. With good deeds that we hope will somehow confirm our existence, that will produce justification for our chosen profession and even, perhaps, for our very life. None of this is wrong or bad. Acting in this way does not disqualify us as health professionals or as human beings. If this were the case, we would all have to resign. But it does show us where our work is. Do you know this place? Can you sense the insatiable hollowness, the catapulting desire to fill this void? The virtual impossibility and exhaustion inherent in this struggle to do good and be needed. Much of health "caring" is based on this sense of helplessness.

This uncertainty, this helplessness, points to where we are encountering our limitations and our hard edges. This is the cutting edge of our practice as it plays itself out in our work. After all, this is all of our story. But it is not the whole story. The continuous nature of this work was transmitted to me clearly by a Roman Catholic priest participating with his fellow priests in an eight-month stress reduction program at the hospital. During a series of deep discussions about celibacy, he said, "I have to decide to be celibate every day. It is not enough that I took a vow twenty years ago when I was a young seminarian. That doesn't work for me today. Today I have to choose. Today I have to decide once again."

Like him, each of us is called to decide, today. To decide about our own slow abstinence from these long-held, reactive habits. About our own opening into the places, the situations where we cannot help. Where the best helping might be doing nothing.

There is a cost for this deciding, for this willingness to resist the impulse to jump in and make things nice, right, or smooth. The cost is aloneness and the slow dissolution of self-interest.

PRACTICE

Working with the Feeling of Helplessness

The power of conditioning—particularly in situations where we are expected or asked to "help"—has an enormous, catapulting presence in our lives. In these moments I notice that working with these driving impulses is aided by my willingness to not act, at least momentarily, and instead to settle into the seemingly inescapable tension of not having an answer, a saving response, a plan.

When I am actually able to work with myself in this way, I sometimes notice that although the sense of ineptness, incompetence, or resignation may have its momentary life, a larger field of vastness shows itself. This "vastness" is neither nothingness nor a disassociative escape but more the feeling of calmness and openness where the crosscurrents of emotion flow with less disruptive and disquieting power.

The next time this feeling of helplessness arises in your life, experimenting with nonaction might be beneficial. There is a generosity of heart in our willingness to stay put, to stop, and to allow these mind waves to wash through and over us. Oftentimes I have discovered that when I am willing to be with this turbulence with no purpose whatsoever, being patient with myself and with the motionlessness of the situation, the right action arises of its own accord. In these moments the breath and your willingness to be still and silent are most worthwhile anchors and allies.

Week Five

THE MOMENTUM IS UNMISTAKABLE. I am being drawn to class by this palpable reality.

Besides speaking with Carla, I have had several other telephone conversations and one face-to-face meeting with a class participant this week. Each of these encounters has arisen, like bread dough, out of the proof box of our last class. Proof boxes are dark, moist, and warm—full of wild yeast—sometimes used by bakers to raise the unripened dough that will, in its own time, be transformed in the contained heat of the oven into a wholesome and nourishing food.

When you open one of these tall, steel, two-door boxes, you see the rising dough in various phases of ripening. It is the same for all of us in class. The telephone calls tell me that some people are struggling and discouraged while others in the midst of this labor are uncovering a growing sense of internal stability that enjoins them to talk about the possibility of "using practice" in particularly difficult situations this week. Some call to talk about the impact of the last class—the intensity of the "work"—and their surprise about entering "a stress reduction program and finding more out about myself than I ever imagined." Still others have called to speak about their sense of desperation, their feeling of a lack of "success" when measuring themselves against the experiences of some of their classmates. Their feeling of hopelessness, magnified by the linear-thinking mind, is convincing them that although we are only halfway through the course, they will "never get it all together in the remaining four weeks." They wonder if they should drop out, if they should even have started, if there is any possibility of working with such a difficult situation, if I have ever heard of anybody in a predicament such as theirs who found "this stuff useful." These conversations often occur about this time in the course.

Following last week's class, because I was so moved by where people were, what they had to say about their lives, and how they were beginning to "see" and slowly relate directly to things via the medium of mindfulness, I wrote a letter to all of them expressing my gratitude for their efforts. The clinic interns, who had received the same letter, were astounded by the gesture and asked me if the letter was "standard," something that I do after every Class 4. The answer is no.

The content and depth of last week's Class 4 has lingered with me all week. The planning of today's class has developed from living with the converging rivers of the sincerity and effort of the participants, what was said, what remained unspoken, and the currents all of this has stirred in me during the week. At this point in the course, we have been alternately practicing the body scan meditation and yoga for forty-five minutes a day, using the guided meditation instruction on an audiotape given out during the first class. In addition, people have been practicing sitting meditation, beginning with ten minutes a day during Week Two and gradually increasing to twenty-five to thirty minutes a day with no taped guidance. Today, they will receive a new tape with forty-five minutes of guided "sitting" meditation on one side and forty-five minutes of standing yoga on the other.

By way of introduction to the content of the new tape, we sit for thirty-five minutes. Then, as we continue to sit, I ask them to listen to a poem. It was spoken aloud by the poet Rumi to his dear friend and scribe Husam Chelebi in the thirteenth century. Translated and titled "The Guest-House" by the American poet Coleman Barks, it is alive and well today. The proof of its aliveness reveals itself in the responses of participants. I speak it aloud today because for them, for me, and perhaps for you too, it embodies an essential aspect of life that can be seen and worked with directly when informed by mindfulness practice.

If you like, read it aloud to yourself.

This being human is a guest-house.
Every morning a new arrival.

A joy, a depression, a meanness,
some momentary awareness comes
as an unexpected visitor.

Welcome and entertain them all!
Even if they're a crowd of sorrows,
who violently sweep your house
empty of its furniture,

still, treat each guest honorably.
He may be clearing you out
for some new delight.

The dark thought, the shame, the malice,
meet them at the door laughing,
and invite them in.

Be grateful for whoever comes,
because each has been sent
as a guide from beyond.

I recite it aloud three times, and we sit for fifteen more minutes. As the sitting draws to an end, I ask people to voice a response to the question: What is one thing you are learning? I suggest that they allow themselves to receive the question, listening closely for the internal reverberations that the question produces, and only then, if they so choose, to give voice to what they are discovering.

Framed within the context of practice, this asks everyone to stay close to home; close to the bare directness of their lives, not needing to censor or shape experience into anything other than what it is. Over the weeks people have become gradually accustomed to this way of speaking. It makes for precision and clarity, leading to the possibility of individual understanding and collective resonance. Although never forced on anyone, this willingness to speak one's truth can be an essential element of self-understanding. Likewise, it is crucial to the development of sangha or community, because it reflects and encourages a collective sense of a group work being undertaken and purposefully cultivated by every person in the circle.

People have much to say. Many speak two or three times. No one remains speechless. People speak about learning to relate to habitual patterns of experience in new ways. Without exception, they speak about learning to be mindful in daily life, about finding themselves in typical situations, acting atypically. Some say that their family members don't quite know what to make of them. Others say that they don't know what to make of themselves. Many speak of being calmer, more relaxed, more flexible in uncomfortable situations. Others report a newfound sense of assertiveness expressed in their unwillingness to swallow what has lain heavy in the chest for so long. The contrast between the anguish expressed during the last two weeks and what is being uttered today is striking. This conversation goes on for a long time.

John describes "The Guest-House" as "powerful." He says that hearing it has helped him begin to understand "the meditation," particularly in terms of learning new ways to relate to the constant sense of change and the feeling of there always being "a new arrival." He goes on to say that he has already begun to experiment with "treating each guest honorably," be it a thought, feeling, bodily sensation, or unexpected situation, and that the poem has deepened his commitment to continue this process and treat himself more kindly. This initiates a torrent of conversation. Several people ask for copies of the poem; others remark about their experience of sitting practice before and after hearing the poem and how it has helped them understand the "how" of allowing whatever enters the field of awareness to be held in an open, noncensoring, nonjudgmental manner.

Francine was on the edge of tears during most of class the last two weeks. This week she has begun to sob quietly, and her unwiped cheeks redden and glisten in this accommodating space. She has faced a hard and terrible loss—the death of her son. Since then she has continued to raise five other children while suffering with relentless depression, anxiety, and panic. She looks my way. Our eyes meet, and I know that today she is going to speak. She opens her mouth, shapes a word, moves her lips, but no sound emerges. She does this again, nodding her head up and down, and with some effort finally says: "How do you meet them at the door laughing? How do you invite them in? I can't laugh, I am so sad, so filled with grief and guilt." Everyone in the room turns her way. There is a collective indrawing of the breath, then an audible sigh as the breath releases.

Pierced by the warm arrow of her inquiry, I know that her asking does not come by way of a challenge. No proof is being demanded. Rather, there is a deep longing to know, to emancipate herself from the undue burden of this reality. It is no different for any of us. And so, I am left momentarily motionless and speechless. This is a good thing. Here, in this moment, there is no room for anything but the receiving of her question. This allows me the space to actually *feel* the question. To simply sense and then slowly gather together all of the aliveness being aroused and released in me by the arrival of the unexpected. Just as the recitation of "The Guest-House" and the work we have been doing together over the last four weeks has encouraged and urged "them" to begin to open and welcome whatever arises in their lives because it is here, Francine's question is the unexpected knock on my door. Right now, beyond any conception of mind, the "guest" has arrived, and I am invited into the possibility of "welcoming and entertaining them all."

Because she has already spoken freely with all of us about her son's death, I speak openly about this when responding to Francine's question. I suggest to her that the poet is in no way telling her that she is supposed to be able to literally "laugh" in the face of the arrival of the memory of her son or of the grief and pain she feels. Rather the poem may be suggesting an inner attitude toward whatever it is that we encounter, urging us to consider the possibility of meeting our grief and pain openhandedly. This is not our usual way of meeting adversity. Most often we resist, retreat, or keep busy. Given our collective penchant, which she knows quite well from her statement "staying busy has kept me from feeling that the pain would overwhelm and kill me," the possibility I am suggesting seems to make some sense to her.

Although the death of a child is not a part of my experience, I have faced many losses in my own life, some having to do with my children. At first these losses seem unbearable and incapable of being healed. I sense that Francine has convincingly created an imagined and enormous fear, believing that she is completely incapable of working with her pain and grief. I do not believe that this is true. I remind her that the manner of her son's death was completely out of her control. Given this, and given the fact that for the last four weeks we have been journeying together into the core of our lives via the medium of mindfulness practice, I suspect that it might be possible for her to begin, this week, working with "being with"—actually feeling in some small ways—the pulse and rhythm of these emotional tides.

We talk about the possibility of approaching what seems to be overwhelming in a way that might allow her a measure of control. Perhaps, like walking toward an ocean in which she might wish to swim without knowing the temperature of the water, she can begin to test the waters of her grief and anxiety with her little toe. Working the edges, not needing to plunge into the center of this emotional sea with her whole body. In this way she might begin to engage this painful aspect of her life at her own pace. Today, maybe one or two seconds. Maybe thirty seconds next week. And perhaps in this way, Rumi's "laughing" might become for her a *willingness*—an embodied, practical way of working with the arrival of fear, grief, and guilt—rather than a running away that has yielded her, in her own words, "little hope or peace."

She listens in silence and nods her head once again. Her classmates are wise, offering her their silent, listening presence, a gift often needed by all of us but mostly undelivered in our world of heart-numbing or advice-giving activity.

Soon it is time to go. Some people leave for other appointments. Many say a brief word or stay huddled close to Francine. They offer no advice. Most simply thank her for her courage and her willingness to ask the question that was on everyone else's mind. Briefly, Francine and I talk together in the hallway. She reaches for my hand and says, "Thank you." I tell her that she is welcome and thank her for her efforts while reminding her that I am available if she wishes to call me during the week. She says, "Okay." We both say at the same time, "See you next week."

Self-Importance 1:
Inflationary Forces

FORTY-FIVE MINUTES down the highway, a short ride to Long-Term Parking Lot 1, then ushered to the terminal by a waiting shuttle bus. Twenty minutes later heading to Chicago. Food. Beverages. Magazines supplied. Board. Deplane. Refuel. Reboard. Touch down. Midday arrival in San Francisco. Twenty-five minutes later dropped off at a new, awaiting rental car. Gassed up. Heading into Berkeley. Wowed! Seduced by the smiling smoothness of the whole operation, the attention to service that has magically whisked me from East Coast grayness to the sunny, green hills of the Bay Area. All of this contributing to the feeling of self-cherishing. The felt sense that "they" had done this for "me."

Traveling north on Route 101. Three lanes moving fast. Passing by new construction. Passing by eucalyptus and dry brush. Moving from sixty to zero in a few seconds. One hell of a traffic

jam stretching out as far as the eye can see. The effect sharp, immediate, direct—like a whack across the back. Sobered up! Breaking
into uproarious, almost uncontrollable laughter, followed quickly
by a spillway of unforeseen tears carrying me into abrupt, deafen-
ing silence. The spell broken. Extricated from the Hype. The illusion of importance.

Traffic. The great equalizer, reducing all of us to enforced stillness and a reckoning with the bare truth of not really being in the
driver's seat after all. The same for all of us that day, whether native
San Franciscan or tourist, driving old or new car. No matter what
our destination.

Self-Importance 2: Inflationary Spiral

JOANIE CALLED ON FRIDAY. She told Norma, one of our clinic secretaries, that she had recently been discharged from an in-patient mental health unit at a local hospital. She's been referred to the clinic by her primary care doctor, who has written a caring, heartfelt letter about his patient, urging us to allow her to participate in the program. I arranged to see her early the following week.

When she arrived she was given a series of forms to complete. This usually takes about fifteen minutes. After forty minutes Joanie was still at it. When I found her in the waiting room, she was flustered. Not because of the difficulty of the questions, but because she felt that she had gone through such a transformation in the last few weeks that she was now being misrepresented by answers to questions that asked about her physical symptoms and psychological states during the last month. In an attempt to counter this situation, she had filled the margins with explanations and commentary whose purpose was to clarify and resolve in some way the dissonance and distance between her sense of self then and now.

As we spoke in the waiting area, her first words were "I thought that this interview would be a time for me to talk with someone about where I am and what the program is all about." I assured her that this indeed was the intent of the interview but that it was helpful for us to have people complete the questionnaire before our meeting. I welcomed her into my office, and we began to talk.

She had a notebook with her, and at times she would read to me her thoughts and feelings about herself and why she wanted to participate in the clinic. She had obviously thought about this in detail. In fact, she was hyperdetailed in her comments. When I asked her where she lived and about her living situation, she responded by telling me about her town, complete with street address and the street address and town of her good friend who would be helping her make arrangements to come to the medical center for classes.

We talked about her stay in the hospital, what had led up to it, as well as her sense of where she stood today. Her comments continued to be microdetailed. After I had listened to and discussed her situation for what began to feel like a long time, she quietly stated, "I'm really here to get information about the clinic, to see what it is all about and if I want to do this, now." With that comment I realized that I was annoyed and that my annoyance was growing. I started shifting in my chair. My focus moved away from her and onto myself. Becoming increasingly impatient and curt, I finally realized that I was being driven by self-importance. I had the feeling that *my* time was being "wasted." That *I* had more important things to do. In short, I didn't want to be here explaining the details of the program and listening to someone ramble on in excruciating detail who might never take the course anyway. I was caught. Do you get the picture?

As my reckoning with these feelings became clearer, I realized that they had almost nothing to do with Joanie, nothing to do with the length of the interview, and everything to do with *me*. I was creating the annoyance. The dissonance. The separation. Joanie was circuitous, nervous, and absolutely sincere. She asked me if she was talking too much. She said this happened whenever she was nervous. I wanted to say yes, but I didn't. Yet her question had a powerful, sobering effect on me. It helped me to stop and begin to see Joanie as a person, regardless of whether she elected to participate in the clinic. As a result, I was able to put myself in her position, to realize that if I were her I would be nervous, and furthermore, that my manner was only contributing to her escalating anxiety.

Curiously, as this shift occurred within me, Joanie put down her notepad, looked at me, and said, "You know, Dr. Saki, all my life I have felt like a jigsaw puzzle with a lot of missing pieces. Now, I have found those pieces, and I'm ready to put the puzzle together and make a life for myself." I couldn't help but feel my own missing pieces as well as the underlying solidity and integrity present behind all of *our* missing parts. There was no reason why Joanie shouldn't have an opportunity to touch her own completeness and well-being. How easy it would have been to make a decision about Joanie based on my agenda, my expectations, and my limited perception of her without ever having gotten a glimpse of who she really is. Those glimpses only arrive in moments of kinship and connectedness.

Joanie enrolled in my Tuesday evening class, and we've had an ongoing discussion before and after classes. The other night she came up to me and said, "I'm making progress. I'm not talking so much anymore." We stood together, smiling. I felt happy for her and glad that I hadn't taken myself so seriously. Doing so would have been a big mistake.

Boxes of Embarrassment

HIV POSITIVE. Turned into AIDS. Embarrassment wants to turn away the eyes. Not out of deference or respect. Only discomfort. Just yesterday this happened. Anna telling me about her life, about her children, about their familial crack habit, about the courts. About custody by the state. About her own struggle to *"recover."* About her desire to live as fully as possible the remaining, up-front unknownness of her future. For all of us the future is unforeseeable, the knownness of impermanence our collective birthright. But she knows and transmits this without pity or travail. She comes to me today as a messenger. There is such a smile on her face. Not big. She knows something. It shows. There is nothing to do now. It is all there in that tiny smile that allows us to speak together freely. Reminding me, once again, of the open, unabashed suchness of human interchange beyond pretense and polish.

PRACTICE

Paying Attention to Embarrassment

Embarrassment seems to come in a few distinct packages. One box holds the feeling of self-consciousness arising out of a personal sense of not having met our own internal standards and being discovered. In this case, the feeling of embarrassment may serve as a useful internal benchmark leading to the possibility of a more awakened shaping and crafting of our way of being in the world. Another, more frequently carried box is associated with a bewildering sense of self-consciousness connected to simply being seen as a less than perfect rendition of a human being. In our relationships with people, this second kind of embarrassment often fuels our feelings of disconnection, because we find it so difficult to simply be ourselves in the presence of another. I was holding the second "package" for some period of time while I sat with Anna. She helped me put it down. Her sheer nakedness delivered me a shock. Startled by a momentary sense of not quite knowing how to be with her, I wanted simultaneously to cover her up and keep my own cloak in place. Then I realized I could simply allow myself to be with her just as she was.

Here are some questions worth asking yourself about the second box of embarrassment:

What is the source of my embarrassment?
What keeps me from simply being myself in the presence of another?
What are we all so embarrassed about, anyway?

The Helper at Home 1

THEY SAY THAT THE REALITY of practice arrives every day, in every moment, in endless variation. Yet within this stream there do appear particular moments—usually carrying with them the accumulated silt of past history—that sweep us into the fullness of our existence, depositing us on some new shore, wet and momentarily breathless, leaving no doubt about the interdependent, interpenetrating nature of all things. These are out-and-out intimations. Fierce, lovingly delivered blows awakening us to the stark truth of our completeness. Reminders of the fact that each of us wears every face that has ever been wrought in the endless tide of humanity.

Do you know what it is like to imagine that you would never again do something you deem abhorrent and believe is no longer in your repository of the possible? Just last evening I stepped into one of those moments. Before I knew it, I had delivered to my wife a tongue-borne blow that totally shocked me, stopped me in my tracks. It was so forceful, so direct and unadorned that it could not be denied. There was no room for excuses. No justification possible. Trying to speak about it afterward was impossible. I did try, to no avail. This morning as I sat in the silence, the full force of the experience settled in. Behind the apology, behind the guilt, the reality of *This too, I am capable of* hung in the air and in my chest. Yet there is a softness about this that is as surprising as the hardness of the initial deed.

Something has been momentarily broken. Actually, *deflated* feels more accurate. What is this? Some fundamental aspect of who I think I am or thought I was has been diminished in stature. There is remorse, but far more present and pervasive is an essential quality of absence. A loss of distinction from all of *"those"* people or qualities of mind that I'd rather not acknowledge as living within this envelope I call *"me."* This is liberating, another blow to that in me that wishes to be set apart from, made special or different from the rest.

I wonder if writing about this is specialness itself asserting itself more subtly. It is hard to know. Yet as I listen to the responses bubbling up from inside me, something plain, lame, and true is walking out onto this page. Some interior wise one who has seen it all, who has patiently waited in the darkened wings, is now smiling back to me a smile of almost unbearable love. Meanwhile, the sun-drenched hero, the one usually walking out in front of himself, separate from the rest, sits down. He is still, at ease for now, watching in silence this old one, captivated momentarily by the light reflected in her mirroring face. Between eye blinks I find myself connected to warmongers, abusers—all the projected *"others"*—their victims, harsh blows sent from and received by me, and I see, once again, that I am not separate. Such tenderness arises from this, that I am invited, without rejoinder, to take my place in the Family. There is pain, and there is a giving in to: a quiet joy, a reconciliation with humanity.

Stepping Inside
the Circle

BEING. UNDONE IS THE WAY we unfold. Certainly, we resist this re-forming in a thousand ways. Comfort is seductive. The desire for the usual, the expected, and the anticipated soon becomes a prison of our own making. I know this in my own life and recognize all too well—in the arising of self-pity, anger, manipulation, deceit, and feigned helplessness—all the attempts at momentary escape and strategic ploy when standing in the strong light of this stark simplicity.

This same process is occurring all the time in the healing relationship. We are always being thrown back on ourselves in the presence of another. Acknowledging the fact that we protect ourselves is meant not as criticism but rather as a gateway into the possibility of looking this reality straight in the eye. Even our style of serving, particularly when "effective," can easily become, without attentiveness, a semiconscious, blinding protection, a settling into well-worn, familiar ways of remaining distant even if the people we are working with do not recognize this. The following is a case in point.

We have a professional internship program in the clinic, and several years ago we had a participant who came from very far away, completely rearranging his life for three months to experience firsthand what he had read and heard about. Like everyone else, he had his own ideas about what it meant to practice mindfulness and to teach mindfulness-based stress reduction. Several weeks into the classes, during a conversation he had requested, he told me, "You are an actor, an entertainer. You're talking *about* mindfulness, but you are not often 'working' mindfully with others when situations come up in the classroom. Your stories get in the way of being present with people." I was angry, offended, and defensive. I disagreed with him, dismissing his criticism as half baked and inaccurate. I spoke with my colleagues about his comments and found out that he had, in one way or another, informed all of us that this was, indeed, our collective shortcoming. That made it even easier to decide that the criticisms were just his trip. But this was not the end of it.

It took months, but what he said finally got under my skin and into my ear. His comments, although not completely accurate, were on target in unexpected ways and had created a small chink in my armor. As with an unnoticed flaw in a pane of glass, over time the splintering began to spread. Did my stories actually get in the way of closer encounter? Did the actor in me "perform" in a way that put me at center stage, allowing me to sidestep the actuality of the moment? As a way of finding out, I decided to give up telling any stories during the next teaching cycle. This practice continued for two teaching cycles.

Pretty soon I discovered that the stories themselves were not the problem. The real problem—the most accurate element of his criticism—was that sometimes the stories did two undesired things. First, because they have a life of their own, they did, at times, create a subtle barrier between me and others because the story pulled us into another world outside of this moment. Those moments were usually "entertaining," but they were definitely off the mark. Second, and far more important, I began to recognize within myself the internal "flicker"—the subtle tremor that some-times reactively brought the story to mind at a particular moment. Often these were moments when I found myself unwilling to *linger* with another in the unknowable, the unanswerable, in the poignancy of a present stripped bare of the next move.

This deep desire to move on almost always robs us of our life. Our willingness to pay attention to this throbbing itch yields enormous understanding. This does not mean that we shouldn't tell stories, use metaphor, be encouraging, proceed, hope for a cure, or use our knowledge and take action. But quite often what is most healing in our relationships, however short- or long-term, arises out of the bedrock of being with things just as they are. This is a long-in-the-learning, endlessly repeated lesson.

Healing is always asking us to step inside the circle, not let going forward or doing something get in the way of being inside this moment. When we step inside and wait, the right action usu-ally makes itself known. Everything becomes clearer; ourselves, others, and situations are seen just as they are.

What Is Shattered?

Men are born soft and supple;
dead, they are stiff and hard.
Plants are born tender and pliant;
dead, they are brittle and dry.
Thus whoever is stiff and inflexible
is a disciple of death.
Whoever is soft and yielding
is a disciple of life.
The hard and stiff will be broken.
The soft and supple will prevail.

LAO-TZU
Tao Te Ching, chapter 76

WE HUMAN BEINGS HAVE ALL become hardened and protected. How else could we be? Bruised by the blows of life, we
have had no deep training or underlying cultural support available
to learn the craft of opening up and relaxing our resistance to life.
What choice have we had but to steel ourselves and walk through
the world, secretly exhausted from looking over our shoulders,

protecting our flanks each step of the way? For each of us, this way of walking carries a price beyond measure. We lose our connection with the world. Life becomes something we do, get through, rather than live. There is immense sadness in this reckoning. Each of us knows this in our own way.

Encased in a no longer selective numbness, we feel cut off, isolated, stonelike, scarcely able to see the moon, feel the great dome of the sky, laugh freely, cry unaccountably while living in the remote closeness of friends, family, and co-workers. Yes, we do continue to live our lives. We walk and talk and glimpse the leaves of fall, but only halfheartedly. Much of the time we live as if shrouded by a thin veil, an internal frost, a coolness that moves out through the skin, rising up between ourselves and the world, leaving us feeling gray, lifeless, and enclosed. It is possible to live an entire life in this manner. This frost, this bleak hardness is subtle and seductive. We are trained *into* it in a thousand ways because it appears to make life easier. More tolerable. Secure.

Believe it or not, in the confines of the heart, behind this stiffness, we all wish for a way through. Melting. Thawing. Cooking. All point toward this work of softening. This has nothing at all to do with passivity, with giving up, with resigning oneself to life as it comes. Rather, it has to do with meeting life on its own terms. As it is. Full-bodied. Affirming. Allowing the heart to stretch forth and speak in its own voice. The voice that is yours! The voice long hidden in the ice chest. The one that still quivers in the presence of suffering and joy.

We are afraid of this tenderness because we think that it will compromise our power, our capacity to think analytically, act dispassionately and directly. Perhaps we don't want to appear weak, unprofessional, soft. But this is simply not what happens. Clear thinking is not shattered. Love is not shattered. What is slowly splintered and cracked open is our sense of personal identification that inhibits the free flow of love. What we call *self,* and what therefore gives rise to *other.* Having a self is not the problem.

Certainly we each embody a unique facet of this unfolding universe. The problem lies simply in imaging that "my" self is independent, separate from the rest.

The melting of this sense of separation does not come easily. It is a lifetime's work that calls for a caring, uncompromising patience with ourselves; trusting friendships; persistence; a willingness to feel deeply the hardness, heat, and light of life; and—a method. Literally, a means for holding the entire dance—the interplay of hardness and softness, of separation and intimacy—in the mirror of nonjudgmental awareness, equanimity, and compassion.

Being in the presence of others who are suffering and who, in turn, if we allow them to, reflect back to us unwanted or undisclosed elements of our own lives is an enormous opportunity to practice in such a manner. Not long ago I sat once again with a group of first-year medical students discussing their initial experiences of gross anatomy. They were halfway through their first semester and had just come from a medical humanities course that through the medium of cartoonlike, self-drawn slides projected their feelings about the experiences of dissecting a cadaver.

The most vocal were those who felt that the timing of the presentation was way off the mark. In essence they said that they had taken eight weeks to stiffen themselves against the stream of underlying emotions arising out of the experience of dissection and wished to persist in this hardening until the end of the anatomy course. They were angry and upset because this had been thrust upon them in the middle of the semester. The crux of their arguments boiled down to this: "How can I learn and think analytically if I now have to deal with all this emotion?" "How will I learn the technical details if I have to deal with charged emotions about this dead body who was once a person?" "Having these kinds of emotions will simply compromise my ability to think and learn."

Others, a far less vocal group, disagreed, expressing the view that this was exactly why the timing was correct. I asked them about their Long-Term Preceptor Program, their first substantial contact with patients. I wanted to move right into the breach where classroom learning and clinical medicine meet, listen to the stories about their initial clinical encounters in which analytical thinking and emotion are joined in the face-to-face encounter with *live* human beings. One man said, "I don't think a doctor should ever cry in front of a patient. I was shocked to see my preceptor cry while hugging family members and children she had cared for who were now being forced to switch to a new HMO." I felt simultaneously fascinated and depressed living inside this moment with them. At the conclusion of the class, the woman next to me trumpeted, "Cut 'em up! Just another part! Later on, after I've learned all of this, I'll feel!"

We left without resolution. Stirred by the insecurity of the situation; opened by the surgical skill, the unerring precision of this dead body. I stayed in the room for a long time wondering. Wondering who had dissected whom. Wondering about education. Wondering about their future patients. Wondering about their feelings of being overwhelmed. Wondering about them. Wondering about the great cultural rift between the head and the heart, between science and humanistic medicine. But mostly wondering what it is within all of us that persists in imagining that we are not vast enough, not substantial enough, not resilient enough, not whole enough to hold it all.

Simply put, it is that in us that feels separate. That feels like a *self* that must be protected. This is the icy hardness. We went right up to the edge of this hardness with no time and no method to enter into an inquiry about this "I" that needs protection. This "I" that imagines that emotion will compromise clear thinking. This "I" that is terrified by the ambiguities, the uncertainties, the chaos embedded in living and in caring. This is not a dis-ease particular to physicians-in-training. This is our collective malaise, the syndrome of keeping the fullness of life at bay while we negotiate our way into a safe, thin, colorless cage. This is what is shattered, if we are willing. It is here, in the slow dissolution of confining identity, that we begin to recover our wholeness.

Ice has its place. Yet when the pond is released from winter, everything is freed. The surface of the water is stirred once again by the morning breeze. Insects find their way to this liquid life, building their homes, eating, and becoming food for others. Plants thrive, waterfowl and otters play in this lithe medium. Water spreads out across the earth to the surrounding banks, and the totality of the world is reflected in this pliant, flowing body.

Likewise, a delicious soup is only delightful because the once disparate ingredients have mingled, releasing a new flavor and aroma. Carrot, bean, or beef cow is not lost. We still know them, still taste each of them as they are. But something more has arisen from their surrender to the softness. In that act each begins to share the essence of its life with the others. When we partake of this mingling essence, their life becomes *our* life. In this way life becomes sustaining, fulfilling, and rich beyond measure.

Being shattered and broken open does not ask us to be blown apart or pounded into submission. Rather, like disparate ingredients, we are invited to slowly dissolve, to enter the pot of our lives and be simmered and softened. In this way we get to know ourselves. To walk with our fear, to feel tenderness aroused, to begin living more fully in the world without so much protection. When we allow this to occur, our burdens lighten, a sense of well-being arises, a willingness to be of help to this world blossoms because we discover that we are able to keep our hearts open and engaged.

Part Four

That's Where the Light Enters You

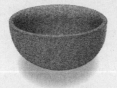

God's joy moves from unmarked box to unmarked box,

from cell to cell. As rainwater, down into flowerbed.

As roses, up from ground.

Now it looks like a plate of rice and fish,

now a cliff covered with vines,

now a horse being saddled. It hides within these,

till one day it cracks them open.

RUMI
"Unmarked Boxes"

Discovering

Radiance

in the Ruins

For nothing can be sole or whole
That has not been rent.

W. B. YEATS
"Crazy Jane Talks with the Bishop"

HAVEN'T YOU EVER FELT shattered and broken? What woman, what man can deny this inescapable reality and still hope to become a human being in the fullest sense of the term? The unfathomable and often dreaded arriving unannounced and unwanted right in the middle of life. The sudden death of a loved one, the loss of a job, the force of a story piercing our well-insulated barriers, setting up waves within us that resonate with the truth of our own predicament, or tales of yet another unthinkable horror of war and human suffering, regularly arrive without invitation. And, closest to home, a sudden injury to the body

173

reminding us of our fragility and dependency, or the delivery of a diagnosis that in one swift moment alters the course of our life forever.

These moments bring with them a power that shatters into a thousand pieces the comfortable cohesiveness, the seeming wholeness of what we call "me." Left only with a life unraveling into memories of the past—a wish for a return to this past, this sense of familiarity—while denying, yet so often knowing, that we can never go back. And yet perhaps sensing, though maybe only faintly—*through* the grace and openness of this brokenness—that like a garden in late winter, we hold within us the possibility of a life not yet blossoming but lying pregnant in the seedbed of our being.

Each of us has experienced moments like this. Our usual reaction is to push them away or to deny their existence. Often we are overcome by fear, paralysis, anger, and confusion. Quite simply, we wish to distance ourselves from all of this as quickly as possible. This is very human. A way to cope. Completely understandable.

As helping professionals we are often in situations with people seeking help whose lives have been shattered or who feel an unstoppable splintering, a sense of coming apart. We are asked again and again by the life arising between us to sit with this, to remain present. But in the face of such anguish, theirs and ours, how is this possible? Is there a method? Are there principles to follow besides the admonition to remain objective and distanced, to feverishly attempt to "fix" the problem, return to the task at hand, or become hardened and numb?

I'd like to share a story that points to the possibility of remaining present in the face of anguish—another's and one's own.

For several years I was involved in theater. During a final dress rehearsal, while perched atop a stack of large wooden blocks high above the floor of a Boston stage, I was unexpectedly gripped by overwhelming fear. My acting teacher, a brilliant, insightful woman named Linda Putnam, saw this fear and said, "Saki, if that feeling emerges during the opening on Friday night, head into it, stay with it, use it, express it with and through your body. First, face the audience and open your legs wide. If that isn't enough, then raise your arms over your head and expose your armpits."

Can you feel this in your body, can you touch base with what she was suggesting even as you read this? Linda was pointing to the possibility that in the midst of strong fear I open up to it, be even more vulnerable, more exposed. She was suggesting not only that the simple act of living inside the fear, and of holding that fear in awareness, was possible but that it might dissolve the accompanying isolation, defensiveness, and paralysis inimical to what was called for in the present moment. And that it could be done in front of hundreds of people. She was right!

When we take up the practice of mindfulness, we are acknowledging—literally remembering—our capacity for wakefulness and stability in the midst of chaos, uncertainty, and the arrival of the unexpected. This is a necessary skill, an essential discipline. Each time we take our seat, holding ourselves upright, opening fully, without unnecessary strain, to this breath, this moment, these thoughts, this feeling, we are embodying our capacity to be present and awake. In this way we reconnect with our basic nature— the truth *behind* the story, behind the momentary activity of the mind. What I realized beyond question that night in Boston was that fear is workable. This had nothing to do with getting rid of the fear or uttering internal affirmations that I was not afraid; rather it involved realizing that right next to the fear was an innate capacity to *be with it* rather than to deny, dismiss, or be swept away by it.

The fear returned on opening night. I remember being able to move into and through those moments. The first flaring of hollowness in the belly and wetness in the mouth, the deliberate internal shift, the turning toward the audience, the anxious throb in the chest spilling out into a sureness of speech and action that carried me into the next moment.

When we sit, literally taking our seat with nonjudgmental

awareness, we begin to recover our ability both to stand firm and to flow more fully into and with experience. We begin to see that everything is in flux, temporal, simultaneously vivid and alive. We begin to treat ourselves more kindly, see ourselves more clearly, and in turn see and treat others similarly. The barriers between self and other start to blur. We touch the brokenness and wholeness of being—our humanity—with less struggle, more ownership, allowing ourselves to be more fully with what is.

This is not to suggest that we can "breathe" or "sit" our troubles away. Meditation is not meant to be another opportunity for magical thinking, an elaborate method for deepening denial, or a means of blinding ourselves to what is before us. What stands as a counterbalance is our commitment, our intention to be awake, and our willingness to relate honestly with ourselves and with others. In this way mindfulness is healing.

There is a sharp, relentless quality to practice and a simultaneous mercifulness. Veiled and then slowly revealed through our capacity to be present without manipulation, striving, or self-judgment, mindfulness practice allows the mind and body to accommodate the fullness of life however it is, with a slowly growing joy and completeness.

As helping professionals we are often blinded by the appearance—the ruins of the person before us. The mind begins to cascade. Sometimes we are gripped by helplessness, driven by the thoughts "What do I do now?" "Nothing else is possible." If, in the spirit of practice, we begin to open into these moments, as painful as they might be, we may discover that there is enormous energy tied up in our desire to escape from ourselves. Practice is asking us to lean lightly into what is, thereby ceasing the tiring game of hiding from ourselves, or disowning large parts of ourselves in a futile attempt to appear whole, competent, caring. Each time we intentionally slow down or stop in the midst of a busy day, whether alone or in the presence of another, it is an act of remembrance of our fundamental capacity to be with, to let go, to open to the mystery and joy of our lives just as they are.

As we begin to do this for ourselves, our capacity to be present with others increases. This is not something that has to be acquired, rather it is to be remembered and actualized over time. When we move into this open space with another, there is enormous possibility. We begin to see an enfolded universe, unabashed potentiality, marvelous possibility sitting before us. Likewise, the people who seek our care start to discover a radiance, an almost-forgotten spark amidst the ruins of bodily pain, illness, and the specter of death. People begin awakening to the possibility of being less subjugated and imprisoned by circumstance.

And when this movement begins, we are turned back once more on ourselves. Our assumptions, our memories, our ways of holding others and ourselves enter into an awareness less dominated by the conceiving mind, shattering once again our notions about who we are and what is possible. This is a reciprocal miracle. An occasion for mutual transformation. Deep delight!

> *Although the wind*
> *blows terribly here,*
> *the moonlight also leaks*
> *between the roof planks*
> *of this ruined house.*

IZUMI SHIKIBU
The Ink Dark Moon

Collegial Sangha

I BAKED MY FIRST LOAF of homemade bread in 1968. It was dense, bricklike, and nearly inedible, yet something captivated me then and led me to work in a series of small commercial bakeries. Several times in my life, particularly during passages of intense change and transition, I have been returned to baker's work. The atmosphere of the bakery is dominated by heat, moisture, endless scrubbing and scouring, and watchfulness. Sinks, pots, pans, countertops, and utensils all require continual attention. Mixing bowls, great masses of rising dough, and milling machines demand constant tending. Baking is a life filled with repetition and precision. Timing is crucial, although it is dominated far less by the sweep of the clock, more by the sight, feel, and smell of dough and batter.

For me, the work of the bakery has always been both humbling and liberating. Humbling because the slightest inattention produces too coarse or fine a flour, misshapes the loaves, over- or undersweetens the pastries, makes them too tough, or reduces the final beauty of a well-cared-for food to the likes of a sloppily placed label. Each time I returned to the heat and ovens, I left a well-regarded professional position. Going back to the world of sweat, to the daily burn lines along the forearms and fingers, to apron-clad encounters with those I'd known in the clean world of my old profession, transported me, early on in each transition, into the unsettling feel of being less than, of having been taken down a notch. In this way baking has always ushered me into the shadow world while simultaneously leaving me a lot of room to work with the raw ingredients of my life.

The direct simplicity of working with the hands, of having before me a job to accomplish, both outwardly and inwardly, has always been freeing. From one point of view, you could say that I was continually learning to be a baker. From an equally accurate point of view, that I was learning to be baked. To stay in the heat and moisture and give myself over to the alchemical mystery of turning and being turned from raw dough to cooked nourishment.

Over the years I participated in the entire process, from milling through mixing to making, packaging, and selling the baked goods. Although I learned each aspect of the process, clearly there were areas in which I excelled and areas that required other people's assistance and expertise. Knowing and seeing through to completion my responsibilities while working side by side with others in a collective endeavor has been most instructive and transforming. Seen from the outside, baking bread and pastry was the most overt, easily understood aim of our efforts. Yet in every instance the most powerful outcome of our gathering together was the transformational effect that we had on one another. Informed by practice and by our combined intention, we shifted from a disparate band of workers to a community of companions bringing a shared vision into concrete reality. This was never easy work. We were continually rubbing up against one another. The bakery was a crucible. Hot, containing, pressurized outwardly; hot, containing, pressurized inwardly. In myth and fairy tale this hot, containing space is often referred to as "kitchen work."

In the clinic we have weekly teachers' meetings for the same purpose. Although as instructors each of us must individually face the undercurrents of fear, helplessness, insecurity, and ambiguity that unavoidably arise in the clinical-classroom situation, our capacity to do so is enriched beyond measure through our willingness to understand and begin to address these issues collaboratively. Because the undercurrents are universal, the presence of these forces is not particularly problematic. Problems arise out of our inability or unwillingness to work directly with these issues.

Our teachers' meetings are a time for us to do this work together. To challenge and support one another. To sometimes confirm, other times contradict, and mostly engage in a deeper inquiry intended to dissolve our sense of isolation and false security by enhancing our capacity to see and be seen clearly. In this way each of us carries our own weight while lending a hand to the others. We call this way of being together *collegial sangha*. Working together in this way is vital for all of us in the clinic, and in a larger sense for all of us in the community we call the Center for Mindfulness in Medicine, Health Care, and Society.

Much like baking, mindfulness practice requires personal discipline and commitment. Yet, because we do not live our lives as independent, self-contained islands, we are always in relationship. Working with others via the medium of practice can be a powerful source of sustenance and inspiration. Our willingness to bring to the kneading bench all the desired and unwanted ingredients of our lives is worthwhile. Our efforts to do so, when supported by and participated in by our colleagues, have the potential to transform our lives and our work.

Just as the combination of solitary effort and collective enterprise when framed in the context of mindfulness practice is salutary for patients participating in the clinic, this joining of work and practice is crucial for helping professionals. If we are not careful, our growing expertise can easily become a prison. All of life and experience can be funneled through and filtered by our theories— including mindfulness practice. When this occurs we become blind and deadened in some way. Although we may remain well regarded professionally, or hold ourselves in high esteem, the freshness and creative edges of our lives begin to diminish as we move further and further away from the transformational energies residing in the raw, unattended-to regions of our souls.

As painfully unwanted as they sometimes are, comments from patients, colleagues, friends, and family members can open us to facing our own unawareness. Our willingness to ask for and receive these critical insights can be a way of understanding and reowning all aspects of ourselves and keeping us honest. In the clinic we take this to be a part of our shared responsibility. This is not simply peer-based group psychotherapy. We are not just looking for psychological insight. Rather, we are attempting to actualize our commitment to assist in one another's unfolding journey. We attend one another's classes, listen to one another's meditation tapes, encourage, encounter, confront, critique, and discuss our individual strengths and weaknesses. Our decision to work together in this manner is intended to undermine our psychological cleverness as well as our capacity to use what we know to explain away everything else.

Most essentially, this way of working is intended to carry us further away from the world of being sure, into the world of not knowing. To be a professional and to not know seems an oxymoron. Nothing could be further from the truth.

Laying Down the Burden of Self-Grasping

The essence of it is to let yourself see how much clinging to how you want your life to be is nothing more than a process of self-torture. Drop it, and allow yourself to fall openly and unguardedly in love with your life as it is and everything in it.

A QUOTE SENT TO ME BY A PARTICIPANT
IN ONE OF MY WORKSHOPS

AS MUCH AS FEAR, helplessness, pain, anger, embarrassment, grief, self-grasping, guilt, uncertainty, and ambiguity are a part of our collective inheritance and experience, they are not in themselves problems. Rather, they are emotions. Emotions often rooted in the seedbed of our sense of separation and isolated selfhood. Being so, perhaps their primary work is to drive us into a fundamental reckoning and eventual exhaustion with our usual way of attempting to walk through this world.

182

If we are willing to be honest with ourselves, we have to admit that much of what we refer to as our shadow, our dark side, or our emotional afflictions arises out of the self-clinging referred to above. In the vast, edgeless domain of the heart, this sense of self-grasping simply does not exist. Yet nearly all of us are dominated by this state of mind in every waking moment of our lives. Perhaps the fact that the isolating, fortified, differentiated feeling of "myself" has no life within the radiant heart is a key to working effectively with this dominant impulse.

Can we explore the possibility that our grasping for the way we want the world to be, and our pushing away of what it actually is, is driving all of us crazy and is, at root, the primary source of our own and everyone else's suffering? Through our commitment to be less self-deceiving and slippery, we may begin to see that this hard nut of self-grasping, of feeling separate and desiring the world to be molded into the way we want it, colors almost all of our lives and shapes most of our relationships in tacit, increasingly subtle, and destructive ways. Perhaps it would more useful for us to understand the source of our suffering, deliberately take it on, and learn that we can work with it rather than attempt to destroy it.

One of my teachers has always been fond of the image of Shiva, a great sage in the Hindu tradition who is sometimes depicted as dancing with a snake coiled around his neck. This teacher interprets the image as suggesting that it is better to know who and where your "enemy" is than not to know, and further that Shiva is less interested in destroying the snake—and all its vital energies—than in harnessing its wildly destructive impulses. Analogously, he suggests that our practice is to allow the "snake" of our self-grasping tendencies to bite us in small doses so that we can locate and begin to understand the nature of this source of suffering and thereby develop antibodies to the potentially lethal venom of the self-cherishing ego.

I suspect that all of us can recall moments in our lives when self-protection and self-grasping have dropped away, if only briefly. Perhaps this has arisen out of our falling in love, caring deeply for another who is suffering, or "losing" ourselves in some other way and being carried into a deep sense of connection and oneness. In these moments the sense of separation and self-cherishing simply dissolves. We find ourselves content, at peace, capable of giving ourselves to others.

Of course, writing about this is all well and good, but we are still left with having to deal with the "how" of making this a reality in our lives, if we so choose. Awakening into our compassionate hearts is a remedy for the quality of self-grasping. The tenderness and brilliance of the heart is an expression of our inherent capacity to cherish and care for others because we are no longer quite so dominated by the confining sense of an armored, isolated, independent self. The following series of practices is designed to nurture the development of compassion and warmheartedness rather than leaving it to chance or lip service. You can begin working with these in your everyday life. I am no expert, but I offer them as a fellow wayfarer and student of the heart.

PRACTICE

Cultivating Compassion

1. Awareness of the Protected Heart

The next time you feel hurt, miserable, or closed down, take a little time and dwell in the awareness of the breath and the feelings in your chest—the tightness, the sense of contraction and the hardness. As you begin to live in these feelings, notice how much softness and transparency exist inside their seeming solidity.

2. Awakening the Warm Heart

After taking some time to establish yourself in the awareness of the breath, recall an incident when you felt loved and cared for by someone. Even if it was a long time ago, give yourself the opportunity to *feel* the quality and depth of love offered to you by another. Dwell in this warm presence, feeling the way the heart begins to soften in response to such love. If you have not felt loved in this way by a person, perhaps you have felt this from a pet. Give yourself the room to dwell in this presence for a time.

3. Sending Loving-Kindness

As you become more familiar with the life of the heart through the receiving of love, you can begin to share this feeling with others. Allow the heart to move from being a receptacle to becoming a transmitter. Holding someone you care about in your mind's eye and in your thoughts, let the love in your heart flow toward him or her. There is no need to force this. Simply feeling the natural tendency of the heart to include others is enough. As this feeling deepens and enlarges, notice that you are capable of sending care and loving-kindness to family members, relatives, friends, patients, or clients, the town in which you live, the place where you work. Notice that, over time, you are quite capable of including strangers and maybe even those for whom you have a feeling of strong dislike or enmity.

This is a form of "practice" we can work with time and time again for the rest of our lives. The intention is to bring us closer to our warm, radiant hearts rather than engendering more guilt or self-recrimination over strong feelings of aversion or hate for someone. Your recognition of such feelings and your intention to work with them over time is itself a reflection of your merciful awareness.

4. Standing in Someone Else's Shoes

So often our sense of the distinctions and differences between ourselves and others is the primary lens through which we see the world. In this practice we can try stepping into someone else's experience. As care-givers, our capacity to get close to the experience of the "patient" is a particularly rich form of mindfulness practice. This practice uses the imaginal or conceptual aspect of mind to begin cultivating a sense of intercon-nectedness.

As you sit with and listen to a patient's or client's story and symptoms, see if you can begin to sense what it might be like for you to be in their situation. How would this illness cause you to modify such taken-for-granted activities as walking, driving, or going out to dinner? How might it affect the tenor of your emotions and your sense of self? Notice the quality of your breathing, the sensations in your body, the stream of thoughts and feelings as you maintain your commitment to get close to the experience that they are describing to you. Notice how your intention and commitment to this process begin to affect the way you listen, the ques-tions you ask, your capacity to feel another's pain, the unfolding of empathy and compassion.

Pay particular attention to the implicit assumptions that you have made about "reality." You may start to notice that the perceived "reality" of the patient is often quite different from that of the practitioner. Knowing this and then attempting to close this usually unspoken gap in understanding between patient and practitioner can begin to shift the entire context of the healing rela-tionship. Once again, remember that this is a "practice," one you were probably not introduced to during your years of formal education. Keeping this in mind may help you dissolve some of the discomfort of feeling you have to perform or be perfect.

5. Only One Set of Shoes

As you sit with another, whether in a clinical encounter, at home with family members, or with your friends, notice that through awareness you can begin to touch the unspoken reality of your shared humanness. In fundamental ways, behind the details and variations in content and life story, you and "other" are not so separate. Do you see that behind the separation something far larger is shared? What would happen if you stayed with the actuality of this shared reality? At first, allowing this feeling to exist and expand can be quite scary; after a while it can become a source of joy even in the midst of difficulty.

Listening as deeply as possible, without comment, to all that the other person has to say often leads us into this domain. Seeing into the eyes and sitting in the shared presence of another is often enough to trigger our recognition of unity behind theory and conceptualization.

6. Watching Television, Reading the News

Twenty years ago I met a man from Montana who watched the news on television and read the newspapers because he said that doing so awakened his heart of compassion. Although not particularly interested in the news itself, he found these two forms of media rich sources for cultivating his growing sense of care for and connection to people, animals, landmasses, oceans, forests, and countries all over the planet. He went on to say that he would sit down in his living room, watch or read about some atrocity occurring in some part of the world, and feel his pain, his impulse to turn away, and, in turn, his sense of connection with all of these beings. He would send warmth and loving-kindness to whomever he saw on television or read about in the paper. He was just a regular guy in his late fifties with a regular job. Big belt buckle, string tie, Stetson hat, and boots. He spoke about this with no sense of boasting, pretense, or piety.

Willing to allow himself to feel deeply, to be unself-consciously moved and opened in the midst of everyday situations, this fellow used a modern "wasteland" to create an oasis. We were in each other's presence for less than an hour, and I've never seen or heard from him since, yet I've never forgotten what he said. The teaching is timeless.

7. Sitting Inside the Radiant Heart

I suspect you've noticed that you can actually "sit" inside your heart while relating to another human being. It is as if you begin to discover that the heart has its own set of senses that allows you access to worlds transpiring behind the seemingly apparent. The heart is both a receiver and a transmitter. We are learning to cultivate and use both of these unseen but often felt dimensions of human existence.

Recognize that you can actually be with another and consciously transmit from your heart a wordless current of care and kindness. In some meditative traditions this stream of care is visualized as green or gold. It makes little difference whether you visualize or simply feel this capacity bubbling forth within you and moving out toward another. There is no need to talk about this or to try manipulating, "healing," or changing another. It is enough to be moved and to silently respond in such a manner.

Week Six

"ELASTIC EDGES." That's the way class participants are beginning to describe their newfound sense of themselves. For them, elastic edges means, "I'm trying out new ways of being, of responding, in the midst of repetitive situations, and it's possible!" Without encouragement, participants speak openly about "layers falling away," about "being more myself," about the feeling of "fragility" in the middle of these deliberate efforts, about being more aware of their capacity "to ride the ups and downs of life."

We begin with five minutes of sitting practice, then move into thirty minutes of standing yoga. At one point during the yoga, we practice a posture that involves slow, continuous, repetitive movement. Somewhere along the way I say that "the posture is never finished," and we simply continue. . . . Later on, Denise says, "This never being finished is so frustrating and challenging for me. I want things to be done, to be completed, and I realize that a lot of my stress has to do with wanting this—with pushing hard to get things done, out of the way, completed—and life simply isn't like that so much of the time."

The yoga is a powerful teaching tool. A metaphor for so much of our lives. Our ability to work the edges, to enter into the seeming boundary zones of our bodies, to be both gentle and persistent in this quest is challenging and points to a far larger dimension of our existence than simply exercising our bodies. People are discovering this in spades, tasting the reality of their own cooking. These are the elastic edges being spoken about and experienced directly. Out of the yoga we transition into thirty minutes of silent sitting. No looking out the windows. No words. Just "sitting."

For the last two weeks, along with our regular home assignments I have asked people to pay close attention to the ways in which we are constantly holding on to or pushing away experience. This assignment came out of a discussion we had in Class 4. I made it clear to them that rather than believe this is the case just because I say so, they must each take this on as a part of their everyday practice and see, from their own experience, if this is so.

When the sitting ends, one man says that he is "shocked" by the sheer quantity of moments he is engaged in the actuality of holding on to and pushing away people, situations, and internal events. Many others nod in assent. This "shock" acts like a call to attention, propelling us further into rather than away from conversation about practice. Some people say that they have begun attempting to "stop," to work with their usual reactive patterns and actually "see" what is happening—by learning to look closely and then "choose"—in some cases, a different way of responding. Others say they are engaging with events and mind moments in the same way. They make it clear that this activity is "uneven"; that the process itself involves a good deal of forgetting and remembering—lapses in awareness—and a goodly amount of staring in the face of long-standing, unwanted, yet familiar habits and patterns, often encountered, before they know it, in the same old way.

It is obvious that they are making a strong commitment to awaken from the grooves and ruts of long-held conditioning. Some people are effusive about positive changes in their medical symptoms and in the quality of their everyday lives. Others are frustrated about their perceived lack of "progress" when comparing themselves with their classmates. I remind them of two things. First, that we haven't been practicing these methods for very long, and this is why we call all of it "practice"; and, second, what they are learning about and working with in themselves are the same things I am working with in myself. I notice that their sense of isolation—of being a "difficult case"—seems to be melting into the recognition of our common experience. What has felt like "mine" alone is slowly being unhinged in the realization of our shared reality.

Others talk about the discovery of "engines," strong driving impulses alive but previously undetected at the frontiers of unawareness. Now they say that these impulses are being seen in all their subtlety as the edges of their vision stretch, becoming increasingly elastic, pliant, and therefore revealing. I am struck by the ways that people are handling these revelations. They have moved from feeling deflated or defeated by these reckonings to feeling, for the most part, challenged and capable of working with them. They are becoming more confident and self-trusting. This does not mean the work is easy. But it is beginning to feel as if whatever they are facing is workable—that it can be approached. They say so. For the first time in five weeks, Francine is not wet-eyed or fidgeting. She is sitting upright and calm; she participates in the discussion, smiling now and then.

Conversation turns in another direction. Gene says that he feels a certain sadness about how much of his life has slipped away from him unawares. He knows that although he has begun a new chapter in his life, he feels as if he's "mourning" the loss of many years. Others agree. Someone says, "I wish I'd done this twenty years ago." A woman with young children says, "My kids should be learning this in school."

In small ways we are all tasting, "taking back our lives," placing our hands on the tiller of our own lives and navigating our own ships in new ways. We are all being faced with the possibility of learning to choose what developmental psychologists call "higher-order responses." We are all recognizing the possibility of choosing more effective responses in a variety of ordinary situations, as well as in unusual, highly charged moments. How this plays itself out is, and will continue to be, different for each of us. Nonetheless, the potentiality is moving from latency to actuality because we are working with a method, a way of transforming effervescent possibility to concrete reality.

I bring a folder filled with poems, quotations, stories, and readings to each class. Usually, I do not plan in advance what I might use, instead allowing all of that to emerge out of the moment. What the participants have generously brought with them to class today, and all that we have discussed, is reflective of the possibility expressed in Mary Oliver's poem "The Summer Day." I ask them if they would like to hear it. They say yes.

Who made the world?
Who made the swan, and the black bear?
Who made the grasshopper?
This grasshopper, I mean—
the one who has flung herself out of the grass,
the one who is eating sugar out of my hand,
who is moving her jaws back and forth instead of up and down—
who is gazing around with her enormous and complicated eyes.
Now she lifts her pale forearms and thoroughly washes her face.
Now she snaps her wings open, and floats away.
I don't know exactly what a prayer is.
I do know how to pay attention, how to fall down
into the grass, how to kneel down in the grass,
how to be idle and blessed, how to stroll through the fields,

which is what I have been doing all day.
Tell me, what else should I have done?
Doesn't everything die at.last, and too soon?
Tell me, what is it you plan to do
with your one wild and precious life?

Alluring and seductive, the last two lines penetrate. Uncompromisingly calling to each of us, moving in under the skin, touching our depths. Everyone sits in the pregnant stillness wondering about their "one wild and precious life" and the possibilities opening out all around us as we learn to pay attention.

The all-day silent retreat will come in a few days. Today's class is almost over, and everyone wants to know what the retreat day is all about. I explain the details as best as I can, realizing that the actuality will be known only in the directness of the encounter. In their trepidation there is readiness. We are riding the momentum of our efforts, each in our own way. People looking deeply into the "bandaged place" are discovering the entering light!

The Path of
Healing

In 1976 my Sufi teacher, with fierce, falconlike matter-of-factness, looked me straight in the eyes and said, "To be a healer, you must be willing to take as your own the patient's illness." I felt disarmed, completely stripped, yet strangely held. Stilled, yet struck like a gong. Drawn forth, yet convinced I was incapable of taking up this job. Then, sitting quietly, he cocked his head slightly to the left, as if listening to something distant yet absolutely at hand. His face softened into a deep, tender knowing, and turning toward me he said, with enormous compassion, "This eliminates 99.9 percent of all of us." In that instant I knew, beyond a doubt, he was including himself in the percentage and that, like any good teacher, he had just escorted me to a threshold, leaving me free to step through or to step aside. In essence he was saying, If this is your Way, then this is what it will take. For a long time I danced around the doorway. I did not step through until there came a rather ordinary moment when I knew that I could no longer not step through. I was never forced, but there was no choice.

In that moment he was inviting me into the true nature of this Way. Helping me to see that this was not going to be particularly romantic, no easy task, and most important, that this was as much his "work" as it was mine. I remember nodding my head as if I understood. Perhaps I did, somewhere in my being. Now, twenty-three years later, I have begun to understand what he really meant. He was reminding me in no uncertain terms that to walk this Way, to do this work, to fully engage in the healing relationship meant that the "I" that I imagine myself to be would have to go. Disappear. Be lost. Completely cooked. His statement didn't leave me much room for attachment to being "a healer" or operating out of the illusion of separation. Over the years I have figured out a variety of creative escapes, affairs of the ego temporarily obscuring the real work. In truth, like most affairs, these have been (and continue to be) fundamentally unsatisfying, leaving me aching with a vacuous, unsatisfied hunger.

But what does it mean, to take as your own the illness of another? I have not experienced much of what the people I work with are carrying in the form of physical illness or emotional trauma. I have come to see that, for me, "taking on" has far more to do with a willingness to enter and engage with someone in the life of what ails them *behind* the immediacy of flesh, blood, and bone. Some would call this soul. It is here, behind the particulars of "condition," that we human beings are joined.

My heart has been broken by the sheer intensity of another person's predicament. I'm sure yours has, too. Sometimes from this the feeling of taking on has arisen spontaneously, without the slightest trace of calculation, out of the vastness of the unthinking Heart-Mind. In those moments there is nothing "to take on" and no one to do any "taking." Yet there is an unmistakable fragrance, a falling away of separation that is at once intimate and universal. The world stops. The passing sense of the present vanishes. When this happens in the presence of thirty people participating in a clinic class, an intimacy envelops all of us. Sometimes we are left speechless, swept into the mystery of the moment. At these times we have all "taken on one another."

One of these moments arrived just the other day. Walking into class I was approached and immediately pulled from the room (literally) by a man in evident, overflowing turmoil. I listened to him for some time, cognizant that on the other side of the wall people were awaiting the start of class. He told me what was on his chest, said he wasn't sure he could continue in the program but wanted to try, and asked if he could shift to another class because of changing work responsibilities and a family crisis. He was relieved and buoyed by a simple yes.

Stepping from the hallway into the bright, effervescent discourse of the room, he sat down near the door just as I was met by the high-pitched, undulating lament of a young woman behind me. Kathy wept torrents, making her pain and helplessness plain for all to hear. She cried out to us her grief, her most private and painful symptoms, fears, anger, anguish, confusion, prognosis, and ultimate sense of betrayal by her body and by her physicians. Listening in stillness, then moving to her side, I waited awhile and then asked if I might place my arm around her shoulders. Nodding, she clasped my other hand; her body shuddered in tidal pulses against my chest. Together, wordlessly, surrounded by a circle of concern and goodwill, we sat, suspended. Whispering to each other in hushed tones intended not so much to hide but instead to hold as precious the raw, tender integrity of this human being. There would be time for other things later.

Later, after class, during the internship meeting for health professionals attending the clinic classes as participant-observers, the conversation quickly moved back to this incident. Although the interns had a wide variety of responses during and following this encounter, with one exception there was unanimity about the whispering. They said:

"Why did you whisper?"

"I felt so helpless."

"I didn't know what to do."

"The whispering intensified my feeling of helplessness."

"I felt isolated."

"What did you say to her?"

"Why did you whisper?"

Being cut loose from the usual moorings of speech and discursive reasoning made most of the interns quite uncomfortable. With Kathy's whispering heart still echoing within my own, it seemed to me that silence was the only reasonable response to them, the only way to honor the gift of her raw and tender pain.

PRACTICE

Exchanging Self for Other

When I was twenty-seven years old, I first learned the practice of exchanging self for other from the Sufis. I have worked with it for years. I am a slow learner, and now, at age forty-nine, I am just beginning to taste the deeper implications of such an endeavor. Among the Sufis, I know of no technical name for this practice. The Tibetan Buddhists call it *tonglen*. The central premise is simple, and at first terrifying to our usual sense of self-security:

1. Touch the vivid reality of the pain as well as the open spaciousness of the heart capable of relating directly to what is.
2. Draw toward yourself all that is unwanted.
3. Take into the crucible of the heart the pain and suffering of the person (or animal) you wish to help.

4. Send out kindness and care to the person or the situation.
5. Extend that wish or feeling to all beings.

There are complex variations of this practice, yet in essence they are all ways of taking in suffering and giving back life and renewal.

Because most of our lives have been preoccupied with ensuring our own happiness and security, the mind has developed a plethora of methods for reaching for pleasure and pushing away pain. In the clinic classes, we work with this by asking people to look deeply into the roots of stress, by paying close attention to how much of the time our lives are being consumed with holding on to pleasure and pushing away unpleasantness. Fueled by practice and the deliberate intention to look into this matter, most often people are shocked by what they discover about this largely unconscious, reactive habit and how it continually shapes our lives.

Exchanging self for other is a powerful way to train the heart-mind to loosen its grip of self-grasping and to know directly that we each hold within us the capacity to participate and work with self and others in increasingly skillful ways. In exploring such a possibility, it is best to begin with ourselves. Otherwise, it is easy to fall into the trap of imagining that "everyone else" needs help but not me. Surrendering to the truth of our own lives is never an easy matter. Honoring who we are and what is actually happening in our lives is the best place to begin. In this way we stay connected with ourselves while directly joining in the shared humanity of all beings who suffer.

When we are willing to open up in this way, not only do we feel the acute sense of heaviness or pain but quite often this is accompanied by an unmistakable sense of roominess or openness. There is a lightness, a capacity to be in this world and function with a less confined and more tender heart. We begin to discover our vastness. No longer having to cling so tenaciously to being armored and closed, we are actually reversing the long-standing habit of self-grasping. Learning to touch our own pain and difficulty without so much clutching allows us to begin to give ourselves away. Such a radical approach can reverse the entire mechanism that generates our sense of suffering and separation. Likewise, because we have been trained to live in emotional poverty, giving away to others our feelings of joy or happiness, of buoyancy or abundance continues this reversal by loosening up all our fixations and tendencies to clutch and hoard what is most precious to us.

1. Giving and Taking with Oneself

Begin by simply feeling the swing and rhythm of the breath. This will allow you to join the various phases of the practice to the immediacy of the breath. As you sit or lie down, allow yourself to make contact with a difficult or painful aspect of your life. Now imagine in the center of your chest a great opening or portal, and draw *into* that opening all of your pain and suffering. Imagining this in the form of a heavy, smoky substance can sometimes be useful. Then, taking in the full measure of this pain on the in-breath, as you exhale, imagine it being burned in the forge of the heart and transformed into a radiant light that spreads through your being. Accepting all of the unacceptable elements of your life into your heart, allowing the heart to respond through its inherent capacity for openness, and then filling yourself with health, joy, and peace is the essence of the practice.

Be attentive to the cycles of the breath. Breathing in suffering, breathing out relief. Breathing in darkness and heaviness, breathing out lightness. Much like the story of Shiva taking in the snake venom, breathing in the unwanted, breathing out refreshment and lightness. After practicing in this manner for some time, allow the phases of taking in and giving out to move beyond the chest, taking in the unwanted through the entire body and breathing out relief through the entire body.

2. Exchanging Self for Other

After having worked with the practice of taking on your own suffering for some time, you may begin to work with taking on the pain of others and returning lightness and life. Riding the currents of the inhalation and exhalation and coordinating the various phases of the practice with the breath creates a more embodied sense of presence and process. Rather than attempting to manipulate anyone, the intention is to take for yourself the suffering of another. Generating this intention, on the inhalation accept into yourself the suffering of another. Perhaps it is someone's bodily pain, depression, or sense of isolation. Allowing all of this to be felt as dark and smoky, and with the intention to alleviate suffering and bring relief to others, send out the exhalation as a radiant, clear light, joy, peace, or whatever you sense would be most helpful to them.

3. Including All Beings

Just as we have worked with self and with a *specific* other, we can extend our wish for happiness and relief to all beings. The idea here is to touch our own experience deeply enough that it becomes a bridge linking us to the rest of the world. After all, every human being knows what it feels like to be consumed by rage, by wanting, by grief and hardship. Becoming more aware of our own difficulties does not in itself lead to narcissism but instead makes it easier to feel connected to another's situation and eventually to a kinship with all beings.

When practicing exchanging self for other, allow your wish for relief to include everyone suffering in that specific way on the planet. At first this might sound sweet, sappy, or impossible. Nonetheless, allowing yourself the room to extend your intentions for ease and happiness to all beings begins to undermine the entire machine of conquest and defeat, of self and other. Although the confining sense of ego does not know quite how to relate to such territory, you may discover the dissolution of its fixed, hard-edged boundaries.

You may never see any tangible signs of relief in another. This is not the point. Our willingness to work in this way is nothing less than the reshaping of a lifetime of conditioning as well as an inherited, intergenerational way of relating to ourselves and the world. It is actually a method of unlearning. An evolutionary self-reeducation that can slowly transform our minds and hearts, thereby creating a foundation for compassionate action.

Vow and Humility

TODAY LUCILLE ANNOUNCED to herself and the rest of the class that she wasn't angry this week. Still and solidly seated, on the floor for the first time, enfolded in a brilliant, floral-patterned dress, wide-eyed and visibly amazed, she looked around at all of us and spoke: "This is the first week in my life that I can remember not feeling angry. I have been given the gift of hope." Then, after a moment of silence, she proclaimed, "This stress reduction is killing me. This is the hardest thing I've ever done in my life."

No one *gave* Lucille hope. She is discovering it within herself. I playfully pointed out to her that despite her assessment of the course as "killing her," she was quite alive and well. She paused and said quietly with unwavering conviction, "This is a start, and I've got a long road ahead of me." She was right, and she had, in her own way, acknowledged that she had taken a vow—a vow to live her life in a different manner.

Vow: A solemn promise . . . to a deity or saint.

Vow: To take vows . . . to enter a religious order.

These two definitions fit our usual sense and use of the word *vow*. Rarely do we consider the possibility that the commitments we make in our daily lives are nothing short of vows. We are familiar with wedding vows, whereby we make a commitment to cherish, live with, and support someone through the ups and downs of life. We know that physicians take the Hippocratic oath or the oath of Maimonides, a vow promising to honor life and do no harm, and we are aware of clergy and monastics taking vows. But how often do we consider that our willing entry into the healing relationship is nothing short of vow? The principle of vow is essential if we are to live our lives with purpose and direction. Vow is an expression of this way of being called mindfulness.

When we say Yes! to serving, we are actually saying: This is my Way—a way of actualizing in daily life, caring for the world as I would care for self; a recognition and affirming action expressing the realization that to take care of self is to take care of others, to take care of others is to take care of self. To live in such a manner demands direction, commitment, and an expanded sense of being that sees beyond the self as a tightly packaged, narrowly defined entity called "me." Perhaps this sounds crazy. Maybe we are neither crazy nor tender enough to attempt to live our lives in this way. To do so will break us open. And yet, if we are not broken open, we cannot really help very much.

This inseparability, this moving into the reality behind thinking and objectifying as the absolute source of information and personal identity, is before us all the time. When we have said something we wish we hadn't, because it hurts someone, does it not gnaw at us as well? Our words never hurt one way. Likewise, our dishonesty and our willingness to be truthful are self-evident reverberations linking us beyond the seeming separation of our momentary location in time and space.

There is nothing romantic about this taking of a vow. It marks the territory of care and attention; it never reaches a culmination and is always an ongoing beginning. It is hard work, always including Yes! and No! as inseparable. Yes! in our willingness to work with and intentionally move beyond our narrowly defined spheres of what it means to care. No! in our decisive commitment to live our lives beyond the confines of conditioned thinking and various brands of socially filtered, culturally constructed reality. Although there is often pomp and public pronouncement surrounding the taking of vows, it is the silent, decisive decision, the quiet shaping of a life unfolding out of this deciding, that speaks for itself. Without vow there is no direction. It is that simple. The sheer intoxicating momentum of life and mind sweep us away before we know it.

We all need ballast, something we can count on and return to for support, something that, like the steadying keel of a sailing ship, keeps us trim, in the water, capable of sailing through unpredictable seas. Practice *is* ballast—a steadying presence moving below the waterline. But it is never enough to say Yes! as if it sounds like a good idea. We must live Yes! This is our work, and it is not easy. Meditation practice is itself the expression of vow and a means of cultivating and acting out of this intention in daily life. Each moment of letting go, of moving beyond the separating, fragmenting noise of self-possessing thought as the ultimate truth of our existence is an expression of vow. In the intricately carpeted language of the Sufis it is said that each of us willingly took a vow in preeternity—before time—to manifest and express in the world of multiplicity and form the oneness and inseparability of life. In the domain of healing, the Sufi master Hazrat Inayat Khan called this way of being *the awakening of the Mother quality in the heart of the healer,* suggesting that our caring for the world is akin to a mother caring for the well-being of her child; caring with no need for reward, nothing in return but the relief of the child's suffering.

This means that we attempt to see everything—all of our

encounters with people, situations, events—as none other than our own lives. In this way, taking care of our own lives is taking care of the world. This is the quintessential element of practice that demands practice. Each moment of return to the breath, to our willingness to open to this moment, to this person, this discomfort and insecurity, and our willingness to move out into the vast wilderness containing these landmarks is a living expression of vow.

Living up to this is impossible.

I am failing at this all the time, having my face rubbed in the truth of this. Such grace! If this were not so, I would be a fanatic or a con artist beyond my wildest imaginings. Being humbled is an act of reconciliation. A way of honesty and acknowledgment filled not with dark shame but with recognition and self-forgiving. Instead of making us feel the need to remain facedown and defeated, these moments, held within the embracing, containing arms of vow and humility, allow us to begin again. To continue on, to simply work the niche in the world where what is ours to do can unfold, can be fortified and sustained by practice—by a method for working with impossibility—lightly, without drama, without the grim baggage of feeling unduly burdened.

This is life-giving. I believe that much of what we call burnout is associated with our intention to be of help and our desire for specific, knowable, well-controlled results. This is an impossibility, sure to generate addictive momentum or sinking depression. There is no way that we can know or make things happen in some completely preordained manner. Life is too compassionate, too wild, too free for that. Our work is to *be,* and from this stillness, to do. To develop an internal stance, an inner posture that allows us to sustain our work in the world over the long haul.

I didn't see or hear from Lucille for a year after the class ended. Then she called and told me that she was about to leave her long-standing job because of the potentially disabling condition that had first brought her to the clinic. She asked if I would write a letter complementing her medical records, stating that despite her attempts to alter this condition, it had persisted throughout the program. We spoke about her situation, and I felt bad that she was being forced to leave the job she loved so much. She was buoyant. Her ballast was evident. There was no false hope, no excuses, no justification or need to explain herself. No regret that she was incapable of openly containing. She said that it was indeed a loss, that she had taken months to come to this, and to the truth about how much her condition was compromising her capacity to work as she wished to and knew herself to be capable of.

She said that she was going to take some much-needed time off, was planning on a new course of study that would enable her to explore a variety of career options and to slowly "go from here." She said that what she had discovered about herself during the course and her continued commitment to practice had sustained her through this difficult time. I felt a faint sense of disappointment, wishing that it were different—that "I" could have made more of a difference and this wouldn't have happened. She must have sensed this, because she said quite decisively, "Saki, this is really all right. I'm living my life, I feel a sense of meaning, and I'm using what I got during the course; in fact, I'm handling it in this way *because* of what I have learned during the last year."

No shame. No pretense. Lucille gave back to me that which she said I gave her. I felt humbled by her courage. Restored unexpectedly by her vow to return again to my own.

> *Come, come whoever you are!*
> *Wanderer, worshipper, lover of leaving.*
> *It doesn't matter.*
>
> *Ours is not a caravan*
> *of despair.*
>
> *Come,*
> *come even if you have*

broken your vows
a thousand times.
Come,
come yet again,
come!

INSCRIBED AT THE TOMB OF JELALUDDIN RUMI

Surrender

THERE IS ANOTHER KIND of helplessness, whose origin is neither fear nor passivity. This one is fierce and intense. This one is full of yielding, arising out of the realization that often there is nothing we can possibly do to change the reality of a situation. This kind of helplessness requires a giving over, a moving into the immensity of sadness, mystery, and seemingly unbearable truth. Often when I am with someone in this kind of situation, I experience this like a long, wordless embrace. Sometimes my fear and uneasiness act as a barrier, and we are set apart. When I am able to walk out beyond the fear, it becomes an embrace that says not "I understand," but something more like "My heart is aching in the presence of this situation. I do not understand how or why this has occurred, and although our conditions are different, I know that somewhere behind our differences, this is also my condition."

It is in these moments that the longing to be of help unfurls like a flag in the wind. It is the intensity of this longing—the surrendering into our inherent impulse "to help"—that does the work of helping, not we. To seek; actually, to be sought by, and embrace this longing requires us to surrender. This is exacting. Disciplined. Unyielding. It necessitates having a strong body, a gaping chest, and a curious willingness to not know. *This helplessness is helping.* It is renewing, deeply restful, full of grace. The doing is in the being. The work is done through us but not by us. It takes enormous skill to get out of the way of ourselves and simply be with another. As servants of the healing arts, this is our *job.* It is a lifetime's journey.

Who is it that wishes to help? What is it in us that wishes to serve, to be of use? I am sure, beyond the shadow of a doubt, that I did not *choose* this path. This way chose me. Does this sound odd to you? Is there an uneasy or resonant familiarity within you as you read this? This does not mean that it is easier. But over the years I have begun to experience a little less of "me"—less arrogance, less embarrassment, less romance—more comfort, awe, and life in this activity.

The impulse to help is older than humanity. I suppose that learning about this used to be much easier, much more a part of daily life. Living in tribes, in extended families, with people at all stages of the life cycle, seeing and caring for the injured, aged, and dying was teaching enough. Caring for Grandma or Great-uncle was just a part of life. In this way perhaps people discovered their place in the circle of caring—where they could serve, how they could serve, where their capacity to *do* stopped. Where serving and caring for another human being ended in death and transition. Is it possible to embrace the truth of this? The thinking mind rails against such non-sense. We have all been "trained" to help. I am not denying the importance of this. It is a part of the circle. Yet almost inevitably this training twists our perception, narrows our sights, and drives us toward doing. This doing is often necessary but always incomplete. Doing needs to be balanced with *non-doing.*

With settling into what is. With realizing that ultimately we are not in control. Life is fragile. There are no guarantees. We are asked to do our best and then rest in the mystery of life. Knowing this can be a cause not for cynicism and paralysis but ultimately for joy, because it is liberating. There is a stark simplicity in this.

There is a price for this loss of control—this release from struggle. It is a great blow to the ego, to the sense of self as powerful, in control, separate from the rest. It erodes our sense of rugged individuality, our arrogance about who and what we are or what we know or are capable of doing. Yet in opening to this, the possibility for deep human connection arises. At first this is hard to swallow. Later on, a welcome relief. Like lying in the grass on a summer afternoon and allowing the Earth to hold you.

> *Nothing in the world*
> *is as soft and yielding as water.*
> *Yet for dissolving the hard and inflexible,*
> *nothing can surpass it.*
>
> *The soft overcomes the hard;*
> *the gentle overcomes the rigid.*
> *Everyone knows this is true,*
> *but few can put it into practice.*
>
> *Therefore the Master remains*
> *serene in the midst of sorrow.*
> *Evil cannot enter his heart.*
> *Because he has given up helping,*
> *he is people's greatest help.*
>
> *True words seem paradoxical.*

LAO-TZU
Tao Te Ching, chapter 78

Standing in Open Space

MY COLLEAGUES AND I often say, "The teaching comes out of the practice." But what do we actually mean by this statement? The question demands honest, open-ended inquiry. I'd like to explore this with you. To do so, I'd like to outline a method. First, I'm going to share with you, quite subjectively, the topology of a recent session of my sitting practice. (This is *not* a model for what's supposed or not supposed to happen while meditating.) Then I'll relate an encounter I had with a patient in class. And finally, I'll attempt to weave together these experiences into a coherent whole. Sitting, I noted four movements:

1

The body settles in. Stiffness in the right knee present and slowly evaporating into a familiar comfort and stability. Thoughts, like schools of tightly packed fish, swimming upstream into awareness. The mind is fuzzy. There are pockets of localized turbulence— eddies in the stream, white water, and small rapids. The mind is scanning. Thoughts appear as bunched, bundled, rapidly moving, barely discrete objects. No apparent rhyme or rhythm, like white noise they are neither particularly interesting nor particularly disturbing. This goes on for a while while stillness slowly unfolds.

2

Seeing moves deep into the chest—literally. Like a huge eye—the chest has opened wide. I know this as the Heart. This seeing is vast. The fish pack opens. There is more water, more open sea between these objects. Thoughts are more discrete. Movement is less rapid. Seeing is clearer. The movements appear both ordered and random. Randomness is more evident in terms of type and quantity of mind waves. Orderliness more evident in terms of process—the way these waves appear in the stream. Everything is slowing down. The eye of the heart is accommodating all of this without selection. There is much room. Emotions are variable and strong—akin to large, slow waves and slower, stronger tides.

3

The vastness of the chest expands. There is more open space. Anxiety arises. I have not recently noticed this in quite the same way as today. The borders of the chest—as vast as they are—are dissolving. The sensation of sitting in the heart is fading from a localized, well-established, familiar terrain into a more panoramic, borderless domain. The mind hesitates in the face of this borderlessness. This is the wellspring of anxiety, the unspoken feeling: What will become of "me"? Watching and feeling this anxiety and the influx of accompanying thoughts, I notice an involuntary movement of the hand, a sudden desire to shift the leg. The mind is blinking, flickering, hesitating, contracting—not wanting to be here any longer. Fear has arrived. There is enough steadiness to remember to "be with"—to establish contact, deep contact—with these feelings. With the turning toward these mind waves, anxiety becomes stronger—a mass of uncomfortable sensations: thoughts, feelings, muscle tension in the gut. This fear is fear of being lost. With continued looking—touching and penetrating this solidity—the massiveness of sensations dissipates. There is fluidity and a slow dissolution of this fear.

4

Dog bark at the back steps, the sound of feet walking on the floor above, the toilet flushing, are now "inside." Actually, there is no inside, no outside. Anxiety-as-feeling-state is present but no longer dominating. Temporary, momentary mind waves including fear arise. Thoughts like "Okay" . . . "That's enough" pass today, without much ado. This is not always the case. There is open space, cool and clear like moonlight on a frozen lake.

Cindy called me about one hour before class to say that she wasn't coming. Too much back pain, too long a drive, too dark and rainy a night. Tonight we began class with forty-five minutes of sitting. When I opened my eyes to the room, she was in the corner. I was surprised and glad to see her.

Tonight grief has arrived in this room. It is the middle of the course, and this is not uncommon. It comes with the territory of seeing and is rarely entered into voluntarily. Often it is accelerated by intensive practice. People speak directly, nakedly. Tales of rage, isolation, insulation, depression, fear, and physical pain surge forth. Together we move deeply into this turbulence, this coalescing moment of life. There is a great willingness, which continually astonishes me. I know that it arises naturally out of sustained attention. Someone in class described this as feeling "plugged in to life for the first time." Sometimes it is direct, hot, like a strong current of electricity, sometimes like the seduction of a moth into the flame of a candle.

People begin to let down, no longer refusing life as it is experienced. The room becomes resonant, each person's story touching a similar chord in another. Cindy begins to sob and speak. "My life is so miserable. I can't get out of bed in the morning. I don't want to get out of bed." We look diagonally across the room at each other. A silence descends. It is familiar. Like the silence before a storm, like the silence arriving at the moment of birth and death—empty, open, pregnant. After a little while I ask her, "Would you mind if I sit next to you?"

"No."

I tell the class members that I'm going to give some time to Cindy. Then, walking across the room to where she sits holding a rolled up green yoga mat on her lap, tied in the middle with a big green bow, I sit by her but not too close. I have no idea exactly what to do or say. I know this place well. It calls for an openness, a willingness to reflect and to allow everything to be just as it is. It is hard work. I am called to listen to and honor Cindy's experience while doing the same for myself. I notice flickerings in my mind—rapid, momentary contractions accompanied by thoughts . . . "What to do now?" . . . "What to say now?" There are ripples of insecurity akin to looking down into a deep crevice that has just migrated under the doorway into the room. Tonight I am not unseated by these reactions. Sometimes I am. Instead, I remain patient and watchful.

We are both standing in open space. There are no handholds. Each time conversation dissolves into silence, one of us finds a foothold—a place to stand momentarily, walking one step closer to where the story unfolds. There are fifty eyes looking our way. I stay with Cindy, and from time to time acknowledge the rest.

"You say you're frightened."

"Yes, I'm afraid because of what I see and how I feel."

She cries softly. I reach out, silently asking for her hand. She gives it willingly. "You said that you're feeling miserable. Can you say a little about 'miserable'?"

"I don't like the relationship I'm in . . . I'm worried about my children . . . I wish I had more control. My body hurts."

There is a long, open space.

"I'm surprised to see you here after our conversation."

"This is better than staying in the house. The house is too damn depressing."

"Are you seeing anyone for counseling?"

"I've just begun. I know I needed to do something . . . I'm also trying to practice. Sometimes I can't . . . sometimes it's helpful."

We talk about her practice. I want to know more about exactly what she finds "helpful" and ask her to be more specific because I don't want to assume anything about her experience. In the telling, she is no longer crying. She says that because she is seeing her life with so much clarity, she has become far more sensitized to just how unhappy she is. Yet she says that she finds solace in the meditation. She says that this gives her a method for taking care of herself in the midst of an extremely painful and difficult situation. She likes to focus on "the breathing," and we talk about her practice in relationship to her situation.

Together, we have now moved out beyond the story. Beyond the drama of her predicament. We are standing together *behind* the cascading waterfall, behind the powerful winds we call "the story." We have not solved a single problem. But how she stands in relationship to the story has shifted. Cindy is amazed. The sunken hollowness of her chest is gone—she is holding herself upright. At this moment there are no solutions. But she is smiling the unselfconscious smile of Dorothy having just peered behind the curtain at the Wizard of Oz. Something has been unmasked, at least for a moment, and seen as it is rather than as it has been conceived. For now, our conversation ends.

Mindfulness allowed both Cindy and me to move *into* the pain and discomfort of the mind. This is not particularly relaxing, but it is often revelatory and liberating. Such a movement occurred both in the sitting session I described at the beginning of this chapter and in our encounter in class. In both of these instances it was the seeing itself, and the being with, rather than any "doing about" that was transformative.

In the face of depression and hopelessness, Cindy touched her pain. In so doing she also touched her stability and strength. This did not happen by my naming it for her or by my telling her that she was indeed strong but instead by the very act of contacting and moving into the feelings of despair and grief. In that moment in class Cindy brought an openhanded, nonjudgmental awareness to her pain. This allowed her to hold these feelings in a particular way. In that moment she was able to see and *touch* her experience rather than *seeing* the world *through* these states of mind. Perhaps this was her first foray into this territory.

The very same process was occurring for me. I often describe practice as a living laboratory. Viewed in this manner, whatever arises in "formal" practice, and how we relate to it, develops self-understanding that can inform us about ways of standing in relationship to these very same mind states as they arise in daily life. In this way sitting with myself and sitting with Cindy were identical. Her willingness, in truth, our willingness, to venture together began to dissolve some of the fear and reactivity. Not because I did any "dissolving" but because this movement *into,* when sustained long enough, allowed us access to the spaciousness behind thought and emotion. Emotion does not go away. But what does occur is a direct taste of this spaciousness. As a consequence, in both of our cases, a reduction or dissolution of strong reactive habits arose.

When we do this for ourselves or with another, all the ideas and notions we have about who we are are disrupted. When we touch our fear and perceived limitations deeply, even momentarily, with mindfulness, we move behind their seeming solidity— like sunlight breaking through clouds our essential nature shines forth. This is not magic, but it is miraculous.

The All-Day
Retreat

IT'S SUNDAY. IT'S SNOWING. I am both swept away and sobered by the swirling whiteness dancing before my eyes as one hundred and twenty of us sit in stillness, gazing out into the gray granite courtyard containing this alluring, sonorous squall. It is 2:20 in the afternoon during the sixth week of the Stress Reduction Clinic, and we are on our all-day retreat. We have been together since early morning, sitting, walking, standing, eating, stretching out into the collective silence accumulating in the Faculty Conference Room, next to the Chancellor's Office, on the first floor of the University of Massachusetts Medical School.

Airborne, the snow, flake by flake, descends. Bouncing, sliding, whirling, yielding to wind and wall, each grain heads groundward, following some hidden Mystery, some invisible pathway, coming to temporary rest—connecting to the rest. Snow on snow. Linked.

Gradually forming dunes and drifts covering in accumulating whiteness the stonework wrought by hands decades ago on the courtyard floor. Today, much like these flakes, each of us has been moved by the shifting currents of the day, and like this snow, our individuality has come to rest—not diminished but both dissolved and expanded into a larger collective communion.

If you walked into this room right now, at first you might be struck by the sheer number of people and the paraphernalia. If you stayed for a little while, the sense of individual "bodies" might begin receding into a vast, unified feeling sense. You see, we are engaged together in the activity of looking deeply into our lives. It is a lively community enterprise rooted in the shared intention to be awake! Today practitioners and patients dress similarly, sit or lie down similarly, practice the same methods similarly. This is not meant to deny our individual roles, to obscure each of our unique representations of human being, or to create automatonlike caricatures. This similarity is itself an expression of our collective commitment, an acknowledged embodiment of the fundamental nature of our relationship to one another. This is happening in a hospital. A hospital contained within a larger academic medical center. A medical center contained within a state educational system, contained within a county with one of the highest levels of managed-care saturation in the country, contained within a national health care environment bent on change. This is medicine moving into the twenty-first century.

My colleagues, Melissa Blacker and Fernando De Torrijos, and I arrive at 7:00 A.M. and line a hundred and twenty chairs around the perimeter of the room, cart mats and cushions in clackety mail hampers from one building to another, rig the sound system, cover the wall clock with a sign that reads NOW, and have a fun-loving and somewhat rowdy time preparing the room for our guests— the members of our classes.

People begin arriving at 8:15, laden with blankets, pillows, lunch bags, and coolers. Some also bring, at our suggestion, lawn chairs to ease back, leg, and neck pain. Others roll out their mats, take off their shoes, sit or lie on the floor, and dig in for the day. Besides the participants in our current teaching cycle, a lot of old, familiar faces are making their way into the room. They are graduates of the program. We send letters to them on a regular basis announcing the yearly schedule of classes, programs, and weekend sessions. The all-day sessions are always free of charge, and many people take advantage of these days of renewal.

For me, it is wonderful to see people walking through the door whom I first met and worked with in class more than fifteen years ago. They have continued to practice, each in their own manner, choosing to give up a day of business as usual and go on retreat. The way they walk in, the looks on their faces, the equipment in hand all conspire to say: I have been here before! They are a welcome sight, and when the thirty of them raise their hands in response to the question "How many graduates are here?" a visible admixture of relief and wonder spreads across the faces of those here for the first time. Given the fact that most of the people in this room have never spent a day of silence in their lives, having thirty people in their midst returning for another go of it is both reassuring and somewhat beguiling.

At 8:30 the three of us return to the clinic offices, briefly review the schedule for the day, and sit together in silence for fifteen minutes. We are also shifting gears, preparing ourselves for this intricate ensemble, for the silence, for a day of retreat. The three of us sitting in the basement, as well as the hundred and twenty people one floor above us speaking their last words for the next several hours, are going on retreat. We are not simply creating a retreat for others—we are joining in retreat. Then, circulating through the room, we greet current clinic participants and the graduates that each of us knows. At 9:00 Melissa rings a brass bell that brings us to silence. The stillness blankets the space as we begin. As the instructors, we will take turns speaking and giving guidance from time to time throughout this day. But we will try our best to minimize the speech by maximizing the clarity and precision of what we say, relying on the pervasive silence from which these words arise to remind us of what our job is and what it is not.

For six hours we practice various forms of meditation, including a long stretch of sustained, gentle yoga. We eat together in silence and play with a variety of awareness exercises intended to deepen what we have been practicing as well as to cultivate a fluid capacity to access and use in our everyday lives what we have been learning for six weeks.

Amazingly it is now 3:00 P.M. The ringing bells enunciate another transition. We are going to move out of silence and into speech. In the remaining silence we ask people to turn toward one other person and *whisper* . . . to stay close to their bare experience of the day, listening to one another, *whispering* . . . We let them know that they can cease speech at any moment, that they can return repeatedly to the silence if they wish—to get their bearings, to remain close to the actuality of their lives as they move back and forth from silence to speech, from speech to silence. When the volume in the room rises, we use the bells as reminders to *whisper* . . . After fifteen minutes all of us move momentarily back into the silence and open out the sixty or so dyads, creating a larger circle where the conversation can continue in the context of the entire room. The discourse is lively and deep.

At 4:00 we silently sit together one more time. The snow has slowed to an occasional flake. Clouds clear out as the sky turns from slate gray to rosy blush. Streaks of salmon, pink, and purple combine with the surprise arrival of the late afternoon sun as everyone begins to leave. By 5:00 mail hampers, mats, cushions, sound system, the sign on the clock, have made their way back to their appointed places. Fernando, Melissa, and I gather for a brief postretreat meeting. We review the day and give one another feedback. These meetings are almost always challenging and revealing. We do not hold back from speaking about what we perceive to be our own or another's strengths and shortcomings. The sense of practice pervades this discussion. We attempt to engage one another honestly and openly in the spirit of companionship and commitment to the work while agreeing that the day has gone well.

Monday we will have our regular teachers' meeting. In those two hours the seven of us will discuss these weekend sessions in greater depth and detail. This weekend two hundred and twenty people participated in the retreat days. Some came for both days. Most came for the first time. Others returned for their eighth, ninth, twelfth time. As instructors, we remain amazed by the thousands of people who have walked through these doors for their first time during the last twenty years and by those who return two or three times a year, year after year.

As we move toward the large revolving door in the main lobby, we expect to be greeted by the accumulated snow. To our surprise, the roads and walkways are nearly clear. The dominating presence and vanishing of the squall fill us with awe and laughter as we say our so longs and walk toward the parking lots.

As I drive home this late February evening, it is evident that the cycle of the sun held so long in the time we call winter is waning. It is not yet dark. Dusk is my companion. Traveling west toward the hills, I am treated to a series of small valleys illuminated in the last light. Although I never quite know what to expect after being away all day, I am glad to be heading home to my family.

The Helper

at Home 2

LATE THREE TIMES THIS WEEK. Twice neglecting to call, determined to be on time today! One more person to see, with plenty of time to do so and arrive home for dinner with my family. His story stretches out, and I have the distinct sensation of trouble. He is disoriented, hardly here, as I ask him the question that I know will sweep us both into some long, winding tributary that we will have to follow for a short time together, and that he will have to traverse longer on his own.

He is filled with remorse and a kind of desperate helplessness stemming from his brutality toward his wife. And he is fearful of the impact of his actions on his young children. She has demanded that he leave the household because there is nothing else to be done. After months of negotiation and attempted reconciliation, he knows that his relationship with his wife and his daily life with his children will change forever. Work has been his survival and his rock. Now this is going, too. He is cut loose from his moorings. It is in his eyes. His sense of place, purpose, and identity has been washed away, scattered in the flash flood of his life.

And I know now that I will be late (again).

We talk slowly. Our voices are distinct yet hushed. He is afraid that he may take his own life. He says he doesn't have a plan, but he's not sure what he'll do to himself tonight if he leaves this hospital. I ask if he wants help, and he nods and says, "I do want help. I'm afraid for my life." After two phone calls we walk together to Emergency Mental Health. We sit together as he is checked in. Like magnets we are connected at the shoulder, each leaning slightly into the other. Then I am asked to leave. This is very hard. We hold each other's gaze for one more moment as the door swings forward and the vibrating finality of the lock sliding into the jamb sounds between us. In the rapidly narrowing space of the shutting door, I see his eyes are wet and afraid. There is a hollow emptiness in my belly. I want to stay. Beyond rationality, I feel that I am abandoning him. I wonder if he feels the same. The tall, solid, steel-banded door closing against my face adds solidity and unmistakable weight to this feeling.

Turning away I walk the long corridors, descend the stairs into the basement, and call his wife. She cries torrents into the phone. She talks of "trying time and time again," of her love for him, and of her sorrow, and she is unwavering in the knowing that her safety and the safekeeping of her children are primary. We say good-bye, and she thanks me. I am shaken and appreciative because I know that the commingling of her sorrow and her steadfast resolve to take a stand and see this through are helping me to do the same. Following a few minutes of night quiet and a long, articulated sigh, I call home. Chalice, my older daughter, answers, and I ask to speak with Rachmana, my wife.

"She's gone to the store, Dad."

"I'll be home late. I had to work with a man who was troubled and afraid of doing himself harm or taking his own life. He realized that he needed help. Please tell Rachmana."

"Is he all right?"

"I hope so."

"It's okay, Dad. Don't worry about being late, it's no big deal. At least he's all right!"

Such wisdom from the mouth of this growing woman. Such sweet, unexpected redemption, going straight to the heart of the matter, releasing me from the sometimes irreconcilable pull of two worlds, leading me out into the cool embrace of the night air and the comforting solitude of the ride back home.

Letting Be

SHE WAS LATE. OVERDUE. He grew increasingly frantic, panicky, as the hours crawled by. The police were called. Unable or unwilling to help, they suggested a number of places to begin to look. He found her on the roof of their apartment building, murdered. He said her last words to him that morning were "I love you. If we never live another day of our lives together, this would be enough."

With enormous courage and a few silent tears, Ted Cmarada told us this story. He said that what got him through this was his refusal to back away from the confusion, despair, rage, and grief. He told us about his embarrassment, about the erupting intensity of the mind grasping momentarily for intimacy with another so quickly after her passing, about the restlessness stirred by this unanticipated separation.

226

In the midst of shock, he called parents, in-laws, many friends, drawn by the necessity of engaging in each aspect of the funeral arrangements—the "memorial celebration." Over the following weeks and months, he took his time, lived in their apartment while his friends and family advised: "Time to move . . . time to find your own place . . . no need to live with all the reminders . . . all the memories so close at hand." He stayed. Listening with other ears to the murmuring of his own heart, he held himself close until he felt his unity once again. He said that, for him, "letting go" was possible only through a self-giving patience that stirred a deep quality of attention to the tiny moments of his daily life.

His telling arose out of the recognition by many in the room that afternoon that mindfulness asks us to simply see, to open to ourselves, and in so doing, to open to the world, learning to be with whatever presents itself. And so Ted was telling us about his learning to be with, about his *letting be,* about his willingness to start at home, with himself, with his own broken heart.

Slowly then, for all of us, this lesson learned over and over again—thousands of times—brings us back to the place of practice. Of being with rather than working on. Of intimacy stripped of willful struggle or internal warfare. Moving into the big space that includes and encompasses the actuality of events. In this "letting be," this "being with," Ted wasn't *trying* or *working at* letting go. His own deep wisdom guided him into this activity. This arose out of his willingness to go slow, to await the arising of action, to allow something to emerge rather than to be imposed upon the fabric of the ragged edges of his life. Out of his willingness to be swept into the intensity of loss and loneliness as well as the gradually remembered trust of being able to stand on open ground— on the firm ground of his being. This is called surrender.

Surrender is suspect for many of us. It triggers fear of loss, of resignation, passivity, and giving up. It is not any of these. Surrender calls for moving in close. Giving up something dear to us. It is painful and it is necessary. Our fear is that we will be lost forever. There is truth in that fear, and somewhere within us we know this. We will be lost forever. But *who* and *what* will be lost—and the concept *lost* itself—are arbitrary conceptions of the fear-filled mind. What is lost is falseness and separation. Surrendering is moving into the center of what is, moving into the spaciousness existing *behind* thought and emotion. All the personal loss, the comfortable, endless dwelling in the drama of experience is left behind, and we find ourselves simply living with the sadness, the open heart and suchness of being a human being.

In our time the phrase "letting go" has largely reduced a dynamic process to a technique—"Oh, I'll just let go." Or worse, an admonishment—"Why don't you just let go?" Can you feel the resistance, the depersonalization, the injustice and victimization in this usage? I know it well, having used it more than enough in my own life. Today, as I sat and listened to Ted, he was demanding nothing. No advice. No rescuing. No smoothing over. Just an open ear, a friendly listening. And in that sitting together, in that opening, that thin slit in the cloth of separation, I came to know him more fully than through any exchange about the passing details of our lives.

There are inconsolable moments of grief that cannot, need not be repaired. Perhaps they help shape the lines in our faces, the changing shine of the eye, the bearing of the body. They are neither bad nor good. They just are. Most often in these openhanded moments, when we stop—when we allow ourselves to be momentarily suspended, fully present with another, with no agenda—we may catch the scent of grace carried from far beyond the ken of grief and joy. After all, isn't this what we all want? To put our ear to the rail of the heart, to touch our own pulse, to be listened to completely by another, and to be, in that moment, known just as we are.

Moving Behind
Personal History

THE FIRST TIME I MET MARTY, he was in a hospital bed. It was during the first class, on the seventh floor in the hospital, just down the hall from the intensive-care unit. There was a knock on the door. It seemed to open by itself, and a bed rolled into the room. Marty was in the bed, complete with raised rails, IV unit, and monitor. A slight nurse with the ease of a race car driver parked him quickly, stepped out from behind the machine, said, "I'll be back at eleven-thirty," and disappeared as tracelessly as she had entered.

The bed was *big*. There was one small opening near the door in the circle of thirty chairs, and the bed was wheeled right into that space. It jutted out diagonally, cutting across the diameter of the circle, placing Marty in the center of our class. I walked over, offered my hand, and introduced myself to him. Elevated and lying there, he leaned forward, looked around at everyone with dark, sad, welcoming, childlike eyes and two days of black stubble, as if surveying his domain from a great reclining throne. Then he settled back and took his place with everyone else.

His presence had, to say the least, a powerful effect on all of us. The distant specter of hospital patient clad in striped Johnny gown, wired up, and horizontal was here, now, right in our faces! Present to each one of us. He was a striking reminder of where we were and what could happen to any of us at any time. To top it off, Marty was young—maybe thirty-five. He was suffering from a debilitating and painful condition in his legs as the result of a severe automobile accident. He hadn't worked for two years.

The following week he was discharged from the hospital and continued to come to class in a wheelchair. He completed the program, and during the next three years I saw him only from time to time in the cafeteria or corridors of the hospital, or when he'd spontaneously knock on my office door and we'd have some time together.

Five years after our first meeting, Marty decided to participate once again in the clinic. He was facing the amputation of one of his legs. I remember him saying to me, "Saki, it's no longer a question of if but when." He was both scared and hopeful. I sensed that his participation this time around was aimed at fortifying this hope in preparation for the unknownness of the anticipated future. Marty realized he'd have to be present. He worked with another instructor this time around, but because of scheduling conflicts arising from his endless appointments at the hospital, he attended almost half of my classes. He wasn't in my Wednesday morning class during the fourth and fifth weeks of the program, and I saw him for the first time in three weeks during the all-day retreat. He arrived in his wheelchair with a big lunch cooler and appeared exhausted and out of sorts. I wondered how things would be for him that day.

The following Wednesday he entered the classroom at about 9:00 A.M. He was in his wheelchair, clean shaven, crutches across his lap, and it was obvious that he had given uncharacteristic attention to the clothes he was wearing. There was something about his presence that was remarkably different. Then, in his rough, bass voice he announced to all of us that he wanted to show us something. He got up out of his wheelchair, put aside his crutches, and walked the length of the room under his own power. People were astounded, and as he turned around and headed back to his seat, there was an outbreak of spontaneous applause.

Then Marty spoke. "You probably all thought that I was sleeping or out of it during the retreat, but I wasn't. I was doing a lot of work. I was in another place during the meditations. And so, when the day was over, I went out to the parking garage to meet my wife, who was picking me up. As I got close to the car, instead of folding up my wheelchair, putting it in the trunk, and getting into the front seat next to her, I told her to slide over and give me the keys because I was driving. My kids were in the backseat . . . they were quiet . . . and then they got real excited . . . 'Daddy's gonna drive . . . Daddy's gonna drive' . . . And we drove to a restaurant for dinner, and then I drove home. It was the first time I've driven in five years."

The room was still, silent, alive. People were awed by Marty's presence, touched by his movement beyond the tyranny of outer circumstance. Not so much because he'd driven or walked across the room but because he'd found himself, found his wholeness in the midst of long-standing brokenness—by *losing himself.* By losing the confining sense of "self" as purely personal history. And he was sitting here today, a living, breathing witness for all of us to the possibility of discovering this within ourselves, no matter what our condition, no matter what role we are playing.

Then Marty spoke some more: "I just realized during the retreat that I've been waiting for five years for something to happen. I'd stopped doing a lot of things because of worrying about

my legs, worrying mostly about losing my leg, about the amputation, about what I was going to do with the rest of my life, about
my family, my kids, and I just decided that, starting today, no matter what happened, I was gonna stop waiting and start living
my life."

Week Seven

IN THE ROOM THIS MORNING, before class begins, the dominant topic of conversation is the all-day retreat. People who attended are effusive. Those who, for whatever reason, chose not to or were unable to attend are listening, questioning, amazed at what they are hearing. People in all corners of the room are talking about what we did together for almost eight hours and how it was both the same as and different from what we've practiced together during the last six weeks.

Sometimes I go with the momentum of this energy and begin class with a discussion of the retreat. Today I suggest to everyone that since we've been working with the theme of communications during the last two weeks, before we get carried further into the current of this discussion, we might begin with a period of formal practice, then look into the connections between practice and relationships, and return to a discussion about the retreat toward the end of class. People seem to be okay with this. So we begin with ten minutes of sitting, move into standing yoga for about fifteen minutes, then sit silently for half an hour. The sitting is absolutely still! When we finish people joke and laugh. People are tickled and say things like:

"After Sunday thirty minutes is a piece of cake."

"Was that thirty minutes? It felt like five."

"After Sunday anything feels like a lot. I was exhausted when I got home."

"Me too. I fell asleep on the sofa at eight o'clock and didn't wake up until the morning."

"Sunday was tough. I was proud of myself, and I'm glad to be back here practicing with everybody else."

The energy wants to move in this direction. We laugh a lot. Banter about how "doing nothing" takes so much effort, hunker down, and revel in the close proximity of one another, recognizing what has been accomplished and how much lies unknown ahead. Soon all of this, at least as we've known it up until now, will be over. Chris mentions this, and the room takes on a new character, shaped by our collective reckoning with the truth of completion. He wonders if and how he will be able to continue without the structure of the weekly classes. He says he believes that he has what he needs to continue but will sorely miss "all of you people." Several people express similar feelings. Someone says he feels that soon it will be time to "fly on my own and see what happens."

There are as many opinions and feelings about the anticipated conclusion of the course as there are people in the room. Out of this mix, Janet takes out her workbook and says that she wants to talk about communication. About "difficult" communications and what she has been observing about herself in these situations. People move with her request and take out their workbooks.

The class is beginning to teach itself. The participants are directing attention to various areas of interest—no longer waiting for me. To be in the presence of this is a privilege. For me, this is the culmination of education, of what it means to be a teacher. People are *drawing themselves forth*. They are doing the same for their companions. I am given the gift of sitting back and beholding this blossoming. I love this. For the last two weeks, participants have been moving tentatively into a more self-directed learning environment. Now they are gaining momentum. I am happy to let them loose from my tutelage.

I wonder to myself what it is that finally propels some classes into this realm. How much of it is me? How much is them? How much is the chemistry between us? How much of it—because I have witnessed it dozens of times before—is a result of a gradually developing sense of power, confidence, and self-trust somehow blossoming out of the duration of the course, the intensity of sustained practice, and the rigor of the all-day session? I suspect that I will never really know, and I don't really care to reduce all of this to a single variable.

There is magic in the room. It's as if all of the *unlearning* we've been engaged in, individually and collectively, is bearing fruit, and we are all learning how to learn. This is no small matter. For the most part, we have been taught not how to learn but rather how to believe, regurgitate, and then pass information on to others. I see before me people learning to trust their feelings, not in the sense of allowing emotions to reign supreme but in becoming acquainted with and trusting themselves in the deeper recesses of their hearts. There is something unshakable about this, and although for each of us it is in infancy and in need of slow, steady ripening, it is nonetheless evident and available. People are sitting in that place, in that seat, at this very moment. Although each of them might name it in a thousand different ways, the evidence of their *presence* is incontrovertible!

And they continue . . . speaking directly to one another, moving back and forth, debating, challenging, suggesting, telling their tales of Sunday and the days following the retreat. Talk runs the spectrum from dealing with bosses at work to sons and daughters at home, from driving in the slow lane to impatience at the toll booth, from the previously expressed feelings of having been asleep to feeling more awake than ever before, from the sense of being lost and isolated in personal suffering to a recognition of what one person calls "universal suffering"—saying he no longer feels "singled out" but a part of something greater, from the feeling of continual annoyance and irritation with the world and with others to a deepening experience of equanimity and understanding. Someone says that "The Guest-House" is so much more alive in her following the all-day session, and that she is beginning to work with and experience that sense of welcoming in a hundred different ways.

By the time all of this surges to completion, it is 11:20. We have not done the body-sculpting exercises, the role plays, or the aikido exercises that we so often use to create a visceral, body-based sense of the various modes of communication available to all of us. Perhaps we will return to all of that next week. Perhaps not. From the viewpoint of the "curriculum," there is a lot that we have not done. Yet we have accomplished what is most important. We have communicated with one another for the entire morning, and we have been led into *communion*. The class has completed itself in its own self-ordering manner. I have done a part of my job by planning for today's class. My planning was well thought out and clear. But that plan simply paled in the radiant wisdom and genius emanating from the people in this room.

Listening

THIS MORNING, standing after sitting practice, moving toward the desk ready to turn on the computer, looking up and out of the south window, I am greeted by blue-black sky and standing, silent sages: white pine and spruce, bare oak and maple. The ground is white, pure, and untouched by feet, four- or two-legged. The rock gardens covered. Deep snow lies crystalline in the arriving light. But more than any of this, I am stopped in my tracks, momentarily suspended by the moon. Behind and above the oaks floats a thin, delicate arc of silver. Now, even as I write, it is turning into a pale, barely visible sliver. This moon reflecting the source of unseen light in this early morning. This sky companion calling me to remember that behind all the activity is this receiving, mirroring quality that gives birth to and sustains listening.

It is impossible to speak, to say what is, to touch the truth that blazes like a thousand suns without this luminous, receiving orb. Why? Because everyone and everything would be burned. There would be no softness. No taking in. No sustaining cycles of heating and cooling that allow for the slow, tender mingling of disparate elements that we call ripening. It is this long listening that gives rise to the sunlight of speech. This moon is mercy. Selfless in its capacity to reflect equally on all beings. Perhaps, like this moon, I too will continue to remember to listen, receive, serve, and be used.

PRACTICE

Listening

For the rest of today try paying close attention to the *beginning* of your conversations with people. Noticing the intention, the first impulse to speak, attempting, when that impulse arises, to consciously *stop* and take one breath. Maybe two. Checking, without the need for self-criticism, the first impulse to express or make your point. Notice what happens in the mind, the sensations in the body, allowing yourself the room, the openness, to receive these internally arising messages while you maintain a listening silence.

Speech

THE SUNLIGHT IS MAGNIFICENT! The sky now revealed deeply blue. The white blanket of snow has turned into a hillside of shimmering, multifaceted, many-colored jewels. The contours of hill, garden bed, and roadside crisply defined. Clearly seen. Big light everywhere. The source present. No subtlety. No need. Just brightness, radiance, and unabashed confidence. Uncovered and present like Michelangelo's *David*.

The thermometer reads twenty degrees. Yet in front of me, just beyond the glass, frozen water is now dripping, turned back into liquid. Freed from bondage. Flowing. Made fluid once again by the very nature and activity of this radiance. How curious that this light also brings the shadow dance. Now I see along the white ground the play of trees blown in the wind, their shadows connecting and parting. Looking up into this blinding luminosity is

stunning. Raw, unadulterated presence. Nothing extra. Just exhil-
arating. Like the moon, the sun is *in here,* not just *out there.* This is
a homecoming. Reminding me again and again of the power of
clear expression.

Part of my own journey continues to be the discovery of
voice. This is radiant expression given shape by mouth, breath, and
deep listening. The remembering again and again of the brilliancy
and feel of wakefulness articulated. I know well that patients
respond to this presence—to the pervasiveness and magnanimity
of *their* intrinsic wakefulness. I ask class participants to become
attentive to the landscape . . . to weather, not just "what kind" of
weather but instead their relationship to "weather." After some
weeks of practice, people begin recognizing, without my saying
so, that "weather" is a reflection of and a reference point for their
own internal biospheres.

This is epiphany! When this happens, everything shifts.
Weather moves *inside.* The landscape moves *inside.* Mountains,
moonlight, dawn, dusk, and sun take on a newness, a freshness, that
is itself illuminating. Thoughts, assumptions, and the play of emotion begin to be seen as passing phenomena. There may be days
or weeks of fog or torrential rain; these states are now seen within
a larger context. People begin to awaken to the reality that these
states of mind—like cloud cover—do not negate their ever-
present, ever-accessible radiance. People taste, awaken directly to
this radiance, the inherent wakefulness of human being. This is
magnificent. In each of us is housed this inner brilliance. This is
life-giving, illuminating, and very near. It must be remembered
and carefully tended. This is neither metaphor nor whimsy. We are
luminous.

The Helper

at Home 3

OFTEN THE CONVERSATION around our dinner table has moved us into the undulating world of social consciousness. We have talked with our children about war, racism, bigotry, injustice and justice, about cliques, isolation, and the possibilities of friendship and human community. It is clear that these young women are developing insight and opinion in this domain, initiating conversation, increasingly taking stands, and holding their own in the family discourse.

Through all these years of conversation, Felice, our younger daughter, had been particularly touched by homelessness, but she had never seen it at close quarters. When she was six we went on an excursion to New York City during December school break.

This was the first time that she and her sister had walked through New York. My mother, their grandma Rosie, accompanied us on our way to Rockefeller Center. As usual, there was construction going on everywhere, and we were forced to walk for two long blocks under the plywood roofing surrounding a building site. Midway through this long, graffiti-painted, poster-riddled gray tunnel, we came upon a little girl—about eight or nine years old—sitting on a milk crate, silently holding an empty Wendy's cup with a sign hanging around her neck that read:

> My name is Katy. My parents can't work.
> I have nothing to eat. Please help me.
> Can you give me some money? God bless you.

Katy and Felice met eye to eye. Felice just stopped and stared. She read the sign, let go of my hand, and just stood there. I wanted to protect her from this truth. My hand reached out and tightened around hers. I began to pull her away. She dug in, pulled against me; then, after a few moments, we turned and walked quickly away. While we all walked straight ahead toward a distinct destination, Felice kept her head turned back, eyes pinned to this embodied reality in the tunnel for as long as she could see her.

After watching the ice skaters, going to Radio City to see the Rockettes (something the girls had yearned to do for years), and having a bite to eat, we headed back to the bus terminal through the gathering darkness of the city. Rising steam, pimps, prostitutes, and street corner preachers everywhere, boom boxes blasting, neon-lighted people lying in the gutters, a cold drizzle, and endless, unfamiliar smells met my daughters head on as Felice insisted that we had to find Katy—we had to walk the same route as before. We didn't find Katy because I didn't take the same streets. Felice talked about "that little girl" for weeks afterward.

Last winter, five years after Katy, we were all in Cambridge for the day. Felice and I sat on a couch in a furniture showroom overlooking Massachusetts Avenue, near Harvard Square. Her mom and older sister were poring over fabric samples as we saw before us several homeless men sleeping in the sun on a cold January afternoon. Felice looked at me and said with extraordinary interest and insight, "Why is it that some of us are homeless and some of us are not?" In that moment I knew that she knew that something inexplicable—something as thin and transparent as the pane of glass between them and us—was all the difference there really was. We just looked at each other, then back to the men in the sun on the cardboard-blanketed sidewalk several times, without saying very much. I saw in her eyes the glint of bewilderment tinged with indignation, blossoming into sadness and unspoken Mystery.

She was connected to Katy once again, linked to these human beings before us, to me, and to herself in a way that no longer asked for the same kind of protection and shelter. Her tender, open sadness was unpretentious, and I knew that my relationship with her was changing. She was ushering me into a new time: a time of allowing her to feel the wind, sometimes sweet, sometimes harsh, blow through her heart. I know this movement well with the people with whom I work. But reckoning with this in one whom I helped bring into this world and whom I have sheltered against this harshness is revelation filled with reverence, slow, painful release, and unexpected grace.

There is turbulence in this grace. And I am reminded once again that caring often asks nothing more than open space. To make such space requires the continual dissolution of previously useful, presently shackling ideas and identities, about ourselves and others, whether we are receiving or giving care. At "home" or at "work."

Week Eight

THE ROOM IS FULL BEYOND MEASURE. Full of people. Full of their surrounding sounds and animated faces. More so, and evident beyond doubt, full of *presence*. There is a collective hum emerging out of an unspoken knowing that we have journeyed a long way, having returned now to where we first began, sitting once again in this circle, yet somehow transformed.

It is the last class. Most probably the last time that we will ever all be together in the same space at the same time. I do not, as the guide, plan this class as if it were the final class. Certainly it is a beginning as well as an ending, yet, for me, the sense of beginning, in all its fascinating unknownness, holds center stage. Some of my colleagues choose to create wonderful rituals as a way to mark this transition. They invite class members to bring nourishing foods, poems, stories or songs, favorite recipes to share with one

244

another. I have been in their classes, and this way of closure is often poignant and complete. But I have chosen another way to mark this passage.

Have you heard the story about the Irish musician and song-writer Tommy Sands, who wrote a song about a moment when he faced that realm into which many of us have journeyed—placing his mother in a nursing home because she was suffering from Alzheimer's disease? After helping her settle into her new room, he found himself sitting with her, holding her hand in his, not wanting to go; knowing it was time to go, not knowing what to say. Together, they lingered in this silence for some time. In that shared stillness he found himself flung by the catapult of sudden memory that all of us sometimes travel, hurled back into his child-hood—to his first day of school. Once again he was sitting with his mother, but this time she was holding his hand, looking him in the eyes, holding him with her loving glance, saying to her young lad, "Good-bye, my love, there's no one leavin'." And so, in that moment of remembrance of feeling his mother's hand held in his, in the nursing home, amidst the grief of life, and choice, and transition, he said quietly to her, "Good-bye, my love, there's no one leavin'," then walked out of the room.

The last class has almost always been this way for me. Long before I heard this story, Class 8 has been shaped by this reckoning. I feel connected to all of these people, some more than others. Yet no matter what the degree of connection, my colleagues and I are willing to extend our relationship far beyond the confines of this arbitrary ending. It is a matter of never giving up on one another. And even if they give up on me, I try my best not to give up on them. People are too miraculous, too filled with latent possibility and blossoming to be given up on. Most important, I wish them not to give up on themselves, just as Tommy Sands knew in that moment in the nursing home and just as his mother knew many years before—no one was leavin'—no one was giving up on any-one else in the midst of a hard shift. And so this last class is shaped by *no ending*.

We begin with thirty minutes of sitting. Today there is no shuffling, no drawn-out settling down, just entry into deep stillness. The moment itself expresses the fullness of weeks of committed, persistent, self-motivated practice. For me, it is a joy to be drawn into the collective silence. Coming out of the stillness, we move seamlessly into standing yoga. Then we arrange ourselves on the floor, once again revisiting the body scan. We began here two months ago, and now we have returned. We have practiced together for ninety minutes. Like almost every other class, we have begun with a long period of formal practice, asserting once again the primacy of practice as a way of living our lives now, and later on, when we leave this room. If and how this way of being unfolds in a person's life is impossible to foretell. Prognostication is not my job, but if we take each day as it arrives, relating to ourselves, others, and the world as directly and as fully as possible, then the future, spawned from this intentionality, takes care of itself because we have taken care of the business at hand.

Now we enter the world of collective speech. I ask people to close their eyes, to form in five words or less, and to give voice to—much in the manner of old riverboat pilots measuring the watery depth of the channel—a "sounding" of where they are now and what they have touched within themselves during the last two months. This does not take very long. Five words limit and sharpen what is said, turning speech into a precision tool. We speak popcorn style, with no definite order around the circle but rather a "popping" forth when you know for yourself that the time is right to speak. Our momentum, containing the gamut of responses, sweeps us into a deeper collective knowing about what these two months have cost us and what has been found in the barter.

From here I pass around envelopes, pieces of plain white paper, and pencils. I ask everyone to prepare a self-addressed envelope and then to write a letter to themselves they would like to receive in the next six to twelve months that will serve as a reminder to them, in the middle of the momentum of life, about what they have touched within themselves during the course and could most easily forget. Quietness arises in the room. The dominant sound is pencil-etched scratching. People work the rhythms of stillness and hand-propelled motion. Sometimes stopping and closing eyes, sometimes writing furiously, sometimes putting pencil to paper in such a slow, considered pace that when they finish, although little of the paper has been filled, an easy contentment seems to overflow. Some write tomes. Others ask if, instead of words, a picture is okay, and so they send themselves drawings. Some ask for more paper, another pencil. And so it goes, until the final envelope is licked, sealed, and stacked in the center of the circle.

Spontaneous conversation bursts forth at 11:30. People speak about what they have learned from one another. About the unusual mix of human beings in the same place at the same time; about the courage, wit, and strength exhibited each week in this room by their unchosen companions. They will probably not see one another very often after today. I will see each of them individually for a closing interview beginning in two weeks.

They thank me for my efforts, and I accept. I thank them for what they have given to me. My life is much richer for having had the privilege of their presence for the last two months. Then I tell them that when class ends I will stand by the door and shake their hand or give them a hug depending on their preference. I offer to a woman on my right the small brass bells that I have sometimes used during the last two months to signal the beginning and ending of sitting meditation. She says she's been wanting to ring these bells for a long time. Now she has her chance! Touched by her hands, the bells send out their reverberating sound one more time. All of us linger in the sound, eyes open, looking around at one another, one more time. For two months each of us has been simmering in our own juices—in our own way. This teaching cycle has brought forth another savory meal. A meal well worth eating.

Epilogue

WHEN I WAS A YOUNG CHILD I remember being stirred by an image of Jesus holding his heart, wrapped in thorns, in his hands. In 1959, when I was ten, I sat in the hands of the great bronze Buddha in Kamakura, Japan. It was a cool day, a dusting of snow resting with me in the great open palms and long fingers. It altered me forever. When I was in my early twenties, I used to slip into the pews of a church where there was a plain stone statue of Jesus standing with his right arm extended, heart in hand, with an open place in the chest barely intimated behind the folds of his robes.

I most remember the face, which was neither frowning nor smiling. There was no sign of martyrdom, no sign of otherworldliness. Simply a quiet presence. Warm, sad eyed, yet full of a quiet joy. Sitting near the statue, I sometimes felt enfolded in the resonant presence of the universal Heart-Mind capable of opening to the world in such a manner. For me, the statue was not a depiction of some unreachable "God" but rather an inspiring representation of love: intrinsic, radical, available, hidden yet capable of being embodied by all human beings. In this way, the standing figure was a reminder. A plain and simple seeing of the human heart that has unconditionally given itself to the world.

The ten-thousandfold impulse to draw back behind the folds of our stiff clothes, our own tender hearts, is always close at hand. In our direct entry into the life of this impulse there is much pain and much possibility. Our willingness to work compassionately with such a deeply ingrained habit is an open invitation for the discovery of our simple, effusive brilliance. The converging activities of meditative practice and the calling to take good care of ourselves and be of help in the world ask each of us to take full responsibility for the welfare and evolutionary journey of human beings, and to put that responsibility at the forefront of our lives, no matter what our role or profession. Holding such an intention and attempting to live in this manner is fraught with trouble and is a cause for quiet celebration. Such a seemingly impossible task is an attractor for hubris and depression, failure and recommitment, contentment and great joy. What makes the acceptance of such responsibility possible is the force of our universal longing for freedom and joy and our wish to accompany one another on this journey.

Living in such a manner is the foundation for a radical shift in our views of self, healing, and the healing relationship. Taking up such a quest holds the possibility of transforming each one of us from cold metal or solid stone to vibrant life. The vibrancy of such life is healing itself, the unfolding dance of an incalculable, ever-abundant universe.

Love does not move us to laughter at the deepest point in its journey, the pinnacle of its flight: at its deepest and highest, it wrenches from us cries and moans, expressions of pain, however jubilant, which when you think about it is not strange at all because birth is a painful joy. A little death is what the French call the climax of the embrace, which joins us as it breaks us apart and finds us as it loses us, is our beginning as it is our end. A little death they call it, but it must be great, tremendous, to give birth to us as it kills us.

EDUARDO GALEANO
The Book of Embraces

Information about

The Center for Mindfulness in Medicine, Health Care, and Society

THE STRESS REDUCTION CLINIC is a part of the Center for Mindfulness in Medicine, Health Care, and Society (CFM) located within the Division of Preventive and Behavioral Medicine in the Department of Medicine at the University of Massachusetts Medical School.

Mission Statement

The Center for Mindfulness in Medicine, Health Care, and Society brings together people dedicated to cultivating and nourishing awareness in the world and in our lives. This awareness, called mindfulness, is intrinsic, universal, and transformative. Our mission is to further the practice and integration of mindfulness, in the lives of individuals, institutions, and in society through health care, education, and research.

To bring this mission into actuality, the CFM offers an array of clinical services, professional education and development programs, retreats for corporate leaders, and on-site programs for organizations in the public and private sectors and engages in research in the emerging fields of mind/body and integrative medicine. For more information, write or call:

UMass Memorial Medical Center
The Center for Mindfulness
Shaw Building
55 Lake Avenue North
Worcester, MA 01655
Telephone: (508) 856-5493 Fax: (508) 856-1977
www.umassmed.edu/cfm

Mindfulness Meditation Practice Tapes

With Saki Santorelli

These audiotapes were designed to assist you in the ongoing cultivation of mindfulness. Each of the tapes explores an aspect of mindfulness meditation practice as well as making suggestions for bringing mindfulness into the daily round of your life. They have been developed in conjunction with this book and are sold only as a complete set.

TAPE 1
Side 1 Awareness of Breathing (sitting): 15 minutes
Side 2 Bringing the Breath into Everyday Life (sitting): 15 minutes

TAPE 2
Side 1 Cradling the Heart Meditation (lying down): 20 minutes
Side 2 Opening Your Heart to Life (sitting): 20 minutes

TAPE 3
Side 1 Awareness of Thoughts and Feelings (sitting): 30 minutes
Side 2 Learning to Embrace the Unwanted (sitting): 30 minutes

TAPE 4
Side 1 Cultivating Compassion (sitting): 30 minutes
Side 2 Loving-Kindness for the Body (lying down): 30 minutes

TAPE 5
Side 1 Exchanging Self for Other 1 (sitting): 30 minutes
Side 2 Exchanging Self for Other 2 (sitting): 30 minutes

Mindfulness Meditation
Practice Tapes

ORDER FORM

Name _____   Send orders to:
Address _____   GUEST-HOUSE TAPES
_____   PO Box 1050
Telephone (___) _____   Belchertown, MA 01007

Telephone orders and credit cards cannot be accepted.

Tape Sets   Total $

_____(set of 5 Tapes) × $35.00 per set: _____
+ $4.00 per set (1st–class postage and handling):   _____
For Massachusetts residents,
   +$1.75 (5%) sales tax per set: _____

CD Sets

_____(set of 4 CDs) × $30.00 per set: _____
+ $4.00 per set (1st–class postage and handling):   _____
For Massachusetts residents,
   +$1.50 (5%) sales tax per set: _____
                          TOTAL ENCLOSED: _____

When ordering, make checks payable to GUEST–HOUSE TAPES.

For tape orders outside the U.S. please send *only* checks drawn on a
U.S. bank in U.S. dollars or an international postal money order in U.S.
dollars.

A Note about the Author

SAKI F. SANTORELLI, Ed.D., is the director of the Stress Reduction Clinic at UMass Memorial Medical Center; the director of Clinical and Educational Services in the Center for Mindfulness in Medicine, Health Care, and Society; and an assistant professor in the Division of Preventive and Behavioral Medicine at the University of Massachusetts Medical School.

He is engaged in the development of a range of experiential, mindfulness-based professional education and development programs and in pioneering initiatives in medical education. For more than a decade he has taught a program for medical students that explores the role of the contemplative mind in medicine and health care. During his career he has trained groups of teachers, nurses, business executives, physicians, Roman Catholic priests, inmates, and correctional staff. He is a fellow of the Fetzer Institute.

His major research interests include the clinical application of mindfulness meditation training for people with chronic pain and stress-related disorders, the effects of contemplative practice in the lives of medical students, as well as an exploration of the dynamics of the healing relationship when informed by meditative awareness.

He lives with his wife and two children in western Massachusetts.